Intelligent Hydrogels in Diagnostics and Therapeutics

Intelligent Hydrogels in Diagnostics and Therapeutics

Edited by
Anujit Ghosal and Ajeet Kaushik

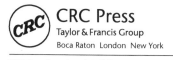

CRC Press
Taylor & Francis Group
Boca Raton London New York

CRC Press is an imprint of the
Taylor & Francis Group, an **informa** business

First edition published 2020
by CRC Press
6000 Broken Sound Parkway NW, Suite 300, Boca Raton, FL 33487–2742

and by CRC Press
4 Park Square, Milton Park, Abingdon, Oxon OX14 4RN

First issued in paperback 2023

Publisher's Note
The publisher has gone to great lengths to ensure the quality of this reprint but points out that some imperfections in the original copies may be apparent.

Library of Congress Cataloging-in-Publication Data

Names: Ghosal, Anujit, editor. | Kaushik, Ajeet Kumar, editor.
Title: Intelligent hydrogels in diagnostics and therapeutics / edited by Anujit Ghosal and Ajeet Kaushik.
Description: First edition. | Boca Raton, FL : CRC Press, 2020. | Includes bibliographical references and index. | Summary: "This book explores the potential of hydrogels as a multi-utility system and their benefits (biocompatibility, degradability, and supporting scaffolds) for a wide range of applications in diagnostics and therapeutics. It also discusses the future prospects and challenges in transition of hydrogels. A wide variety of smart hydrogels (conducting, stimuli-responsive, and others) with possible biomedical applications have been elaborated. The book demonstrates the effectiveness of hydrogels in diagnostics of diseases in various in-vivo and in-vitro environments and highlights the designing with engineering/functionalization of hydrogels for everyday drug dosage as an efficient drug carrier, scaffold and sensing application" — Provided by publisher.
Identifiers: LCCN 2019058115 | ISBN 9781138361218 (hardback) | ISBN 9781003036050 (ebook)
Subjects: LCSH: Colloids in medicine. | Colloids—Biotechnology.
Classification: LCC R857.C66 I58 2020 | DDC 610.28—dc23
LC record available at https://lccn.loc.gov/2019058115

ISBN-13: 978-1-138-36121-8 (hbk)
ISBN-13: 978-1-03-265355-6 (pbk)
ISBN-13: 978-1-00-303605-0 (ebk)

DOI: 10.1201/9781003036050

Typeset in Times
by Apex CoVantage, LLC

Contents

Tanya Chhibber, Ravikumar Shinde, Behnaz Lahooti,
Sounak Bagchi, Sree Pooja Varahachalam, Anusha
Gaddam, Amit K. Jaiswal, Evelyn Gracia, Hitendra
S. Chand, Ajeet Kaushik, and Rahul Dev Jayant

Jyoti Bala, Anupam J. Das, and Ajeet Kaushik

Arti Vashist, Rameen Walters, and Madhavan Nair

Contents

ix

Preface

Nanotechnology has been affecting the scientific arenas and has particularly revolutionized the field of health care. Growth in nanobiotechnology influences drug delivery, diagnostics, and therapeutics. On-demand delivery and continuous controlled release improve the efficacy as well as lower the toxicity of any drug. Achieving such perfection in the field of theranostics would be guided by the development of tunable and functionalized hydrogel systems.

This book explores the interdisciplinary aspect of nanotechnology, chemistry, and biology. The potential of hydrogels as a multiutility system and their benefits (biocompatibility, degradability, and supporting scaffolds) for a wide range of applications have been highlighted. Fabrication of such biotheranostic agents and possible variations have improved the delivery of the product and the antibacterial activity and targeting behavior of the gel system. The challenges and future of such systems with transitional benefits associated with nanogels have been also projected. The projected salient features of the book are expressed as follows.

- Explores the prospects of nanobiotechnology in development of medicinal utilities in the health care industry
- Highlights the designing and engineering of hydrogels for required everyday drug dosage and possible functionalization to fabricate an efficient drug carrier
- Covers the significance of biopolymer-based hydrogels and their responsiveness in different physiological fluids
- Demonstrates the effectiveness in diagnostics of diseases in various in vivo and in vitro environments
- Seeds new ideas in the development of novel and next-generation theranostics units
- Discusses the prospects and challenges in the transition from hydrogels to nanogels

The medicinal value of many drugs can be enhanced greatly provided they are delivered by using an efficient delivery mechanism and carrier. In this regard, hydrogels can be one of the potential candidates which can be utilized in different modes, ranging from diagnosis to therapeutics as a personalized Medicare unit.

This book discusses the mechanistic aspect of synthesis and designing as per the application of hydrogels. Apart from general biomedical applications, the aspect and benefits of using hydrogels for diagnosis along with simultaneous therapeutic ability have been highlighted with case studies. Apart from various biomedical applications like drug delivery, tissue engineering, biosensor design, and type of polymers used, the book projects the importance of polymeric hydrogels and nano-based interalterations. Responsiveness under varied environments and theranostic ability of the cross-linked polymeric material has been presented. Additional information regarding the use of hydrogels, the value-added properties on the introduction of magnetic properties and nanofillers, and the present challenges and prospects in the fields of drug delivery, biomedical applications, and therapeutics have been elaborated. The section related to magnetic hydrogels and their specific use for targeted drug delivery, imaging and highlights about various key designing tips in the prospects of the book increases the novelty. The covered chapters with a brief description are summarized here.

1. *Hydrogels and their fundamentals:* A brief overview of the journey of hydrogels and various classes of hydrogels available for medical applications are presented. The properties and improvement in respective abilities through the application of nanotechnology as a biomedical resource are discussed.

2. *Role of nanobiotechnology in hydrogels and their medicinal advancements:* The importance of hydrogels, interpenetrating networked hydrogels, and nanogels with the effect of nanotechnology on adsorption, scaffold, tissue engineering, and DNA hydrogels are discussed. The discussion of the possible required material for such application and role of nanotechnology is elaborated.

3. *Conducting polymer-based hydrogels and scaffolds:* The role of conductivity in hydrogels for various biomedical purposes is elaborated. The use of conducting polymers (polyaniline, polypyrrole, and polythiophene) in hydrogels and their unique properties in tissue engineering/drug delivery and other biomedical applications are presented.

4. *Smart hydrogels and their responsiveness:* How the chemical composition and cross-linking of individual components alters the response of designed hydrogels under different environments. The exploitation of this ability in the development of stimuli-responsive drug delivery agents is described with case studies and future perspectives.

5. *Hydrogel for sensing application:* Hydrogels and the mechanism of sensing ability of the same are elaborated. Sensitivity based on molecular interaction, bacteria, cells, and other variations in the chemical or physical environment is explained.

6. *Biomedical application of hydrogel and their importance:* Brief classification of hydrogels with the general application of hydrogels is explained. Different drug delivery (diffusion, chemically, and swelling controlled) mechanisms are presented along with other biomedical applications of hydrogels.

7. *Hydrogels and their imaging application:* Introduction to smart hydrogels and their imaging application. The importance of imaging for guided therapeutics in tumor detection, intercellular imaging, tissue engineering, and sensing application is presented.

8. *Hydrogels in tissue engineering:* The chapter discusses the naturally active scaffolds, basic synthesis process, and their applications in tissue engineering. Limitations, challenges, and future aspects of clinical applications are also discussed.

9. *Antibacterial hydrogels and their implications:* Additional ability of pre-designed hydrogels for their prospective use as antibacterial material

for coating and other implications. Hydrogels with inherent antimicrobial activity and nanoparticle incorporated hydrogels for the application are discussed.

10. ***Challenges and future prospects associated with smart hydrogels for drug delivery and imaging:*** Upcoming prospects, present challenges associated with hydrogels, and possible in-hand limitations are discussed at length.

This book is an attempt to describe the need, mechanisms, growth, and application of novel hydrogels in combination with the impact of nanobiotechnology. Thus, potential multifaceted applications of smart hydrogels along with recent advancements in this field have been majorly highlighted through different chapters. The bifurcation is intended to bridge an understanding between theranostics aspects of intelligent hydrogels.

This book will provide an overview of the role of nanobiotechnology in developing advances as well as multifunction delivery cum diagnostic systems for health care and personalized health benefits.

Anujit Ghosal, Ph.D.
School of Biotechnology
Jawaharlal Nehru University
and
School of Life Sciences
Beijing Institute of Technology
Beijing, PRC

Ajeet Kaushik, Ph.D.
Department of Natural Sciences,
Florida Polytechnic University
Lakeland, US

Editor Biographies

At present, **Dr. Anujit Ghosal** is associated with the School of Life Science in Beijing Institute of Technology, Beijing, PRC. Previously, he has been a recipient of the prestigious National Postdoctoral Fellowship at the School of Biotechnology, Jawaharlal Nehru University, New Delhi, India. He has worked on three-dimensional hydrogels for drug delivery, cell culture, and biomedical applications. Additionally, he has worked on the preparation of inorganic-organic hybrid materials using synthetic and biopolymers for development of surface protective coatings/films. He has also worked as an assistant professor for chemistry at Galgotias University, India.

His research ability is proven by his published peer-reviewed research articles in journals of high repute, review articles, and contributed book chapters. His area of research involves mostly hydrogels, catalysis, biosensors, electrochemistry, corrosion, and fabrication of nanomaterials for possible biomedical applications.

Dr. Ajeet Kaushik received his Ph.D. (chemistry, biosensors; 2010) in collaboration with the National Physical Laboratory and Jamia Milia Islamia, New Delhi, India. Presently, Dr. Kaushik, as an assistant professor of chemistry, is exploring advanced electrochemical sensing systems and nanomedicine for personalized health wellness at the Department of Natural Sciences of the Division of Science, Arts, and Mathematics at Florida Polytechnic University, Lakeland, US. He is the recipient of various reputed awards for his service in the area of nanobiotechnology for health care. His excellent research credentials are reflected by his four edited books, 100 international research peer-reviewed publications, and three patents in the area of nanomedicine and smart biosensors for personalized health care. In the course of his research, Dr. Kaushik has been engaged in design and development of various electroactive nanostructures for electrochemical biosensors and nanomedicine for health care. His research interests include nanobiotechnology, analytical systems, design and development of nanostructures, nanocarries for drug delivery, nanotherapeutics for CNS diseases, on-demand site-specific release of therapeutic agents, exploring personalized nanomedicines, biosensors, point-of-care sensing devices, and related areas of health care monitoring.

Contributors

Eijaz Ahmed Bhat, Ph.D.
Life Science Institute,
Zhejiang University,
Hangzhou, Zhejiang, China

Muhammad Arsalan, Ph.D.
College of Chemistry and
Materials Science,
Northwest University, Xi'an, China

Sounak Bagchi
Department of Pharmaceutical
Sciences, School of Pharmacy,
Texas Tech University Health
Sciences Center,
Amarillo, TX, US

Jyoti Bala
Department of Natural Sciences,
Division of Science, Arts,
and Mathematics (SAM),
Florida Polytechnic University,
Lakeland, FL, US

Suryasarathi Bose, Ph.D.
Department of Materials Engineering,
Indian Institute of Science,
Bangalore, India

Hitendra S. Chand
Department of Immunology and
Nano-Medicine,
Herbert Wertheim College of Medicine,
Florida International University (FIU),
Miami, FL, US

Tanya Chhibber, M.S.
Department of Pharmaceutical
Sciences, School of Pharmacy,
Texas Tech University Health
Sciences Center,
Amarillo, TX, US

Anupam J. Das
Department of Natural Sciences,
Division of Science, Arts,
and Mathematics (SAM),
Florida Polytechnic University,
Lakeland, FL, US

Tarun Kumar Dhiman
Special Centre for Nanoscience,
Jawaharlal Nehru University,
New Delhi, India

Rupak Dua
Department of Chemical Engineering,
Hampton University,
Hampton, Virginia, US

Anusha Gaddam
Department of Pharmaceutical
Sciences, School of Pharmacy,
Texas Tech University Health
Sciences Center,
Amarillo, TX, US

Anujit Ghosal
School of Life Science,
Beijing Institute of Technology,
Beijing, China
School of Biotechnology,
Jawaharlal Nehru University,
New Delhi, India

Evelyn Gracia
Department of Immunology and Nano-
Medicine,
Herbert Wertheim College of
Medicine,
Florida International
University (FIU),
Miami, FL, US

Amit K. Jaiswal
School of Biosciences and
    Biotechnology (SBST),
    Vellore Institute of
    Technology (VIT),
    Vellore, Tamilnadu, India

Rahul Dev Jayant, Ph.D.
Department of Pharmaceutical
    Sciences, School of Pharmacy,
    Texas Tech University Health
    Sciences Center,
    Amarillo, TX, US

Ajeet Kaushik, Ph.D.
Department of Natural Sciences,
    Division of Science, Arts,
    and Mathematics (SAM),
    Florida Polytechnic University,
    Lakeland, FL, US

Behnaz Lahooti
Department of Pharmaceutical
    Sciences, School of Pharmacy,
    Texas Tech University Health
    Sciences Center,
    Amarillo, TX, US

Ifrah Manzoor
Department of Biochemistry,
    University of Kashmir,
    Hazratbal, Srinagar, India

Abhijeet Mishra, Ph.D.
Acharya Narendra Dev College,
    University of Delhi, New
    Delhi, India

Madhavan Nair, Ph.D.
Center for Personalized
    Nanomedicine, Institute of
    NeuroImmune Pharmacology,
    Department of Immunology
    and Nano-Medicine,
    Herbert Wertheim College of Medicine,
    Florida International University,
    Miami, FL, US

Wasifa Noor
Centre of Research for Development,
    University of Kashmir,
    Hazratbal, Srinagar, India

Shabnam Pathan, Ph.D.
Department of Materials
    Engineering, Indian Institute of
    Science,
    Bangalore, India

Rangnath Ravi
Department of Chemistry, Jamia
    Millia Islamia,
    New Delhi, India

Neha Kanwar Rawat, Ph.D.
Materials Science Division, CSIR-
    National Aerospace Laboratories,
    Bengaluru,
    Karnataka, India

Nasreena Sajjad, Ph.D.
Department of Biochemistry,
    University of Kashmir,
    Hazratbal, Srinagar, India

Tamal Sarkar, Ph.D.
Special Centre for Nanoscience,
    Jawaharlal Nehru University,
    New Delhi, India

Durdana Shah
Centre of Research for Development,
    University of Kashmir,
    Hazratbal, Srinagar, India

Shumaila Shaukat, Ph.D.
College of Chemistry and Materials
    Science,
    Northwest University,
    Xi'an, China

Ravikumar Shinde
Rajarshi Shahu Mahavidyalaya,
    Latur, Maharashtra, India

Namita Singh
Department of Biomedical Science,
    Acharya Narendra Dev College,
    University of Delhi,
    New Delhi, India

Partima R. Solanki
Special Centre for Nanoscience,
    Jawaharlal Nehru University,
    New Delhi, India

Darryl Taylor
Department of Chemical
    Engineering, Hampton
    University,
    Hampton, Virginia, US

Sree Pooja Varahachalam
Department of Pharmaceutical
    Sciences, School of Pharmacy,
    Texas Tech University Health
    Sciences Center,
    Amarillo, TX, US

Arti Vashist
Center for Personalized
    Nanomedicine, Institute of
    NeuroImmune Pharmacology,
    Department of Immunology and
    Nano-Medicine, Herbert Wertheim
    College of Medicine,
    Florida International University,
    Miami, FL, US

Rameen Walters
Center for Personalized
    Nanomedicine, Institute of
    NeuroImmune Pharmacology,
    Department of Immunology and
    Nano-Medicine, Herbert Wertheim
    College of Medicine,
    Florida International University,
    Miami, FL, US

Yinmao Wei
College of Chemistry and Materials Science,
    Northwest University,
    Xi'an, China

1 Hydrogels and Their Fundamentals

Shabnam Pathan and Suryasarathi Bose

CONTENTS

1.1 HYDROGELS

The name 'hydrogel' was first coined in the year 1894, when it was called a colloidal gel of inorganic salts. Afterward, subsequent development in this field led to many discoveries and innovations. At initial stages, cross-linked PVA hydrogel was fabricated by gamma irradiation in 1958. Wichterle and Lim introduced hydrogels for contact lens application using poly (HEMA) in 1960 and so forth [1–3].

Hydrogels are highly cross-linked three-dimensional network structures capable of absorbing huge amount of water because of the presence of polar groups like carboxyl, hydroxyl, amide, sulphonic groups. Hydrogels are held together by either physical interactions or chemical cross-links. With variation in the extent of highly cross-linked network structure, hydrogels show different degrees of swelling behavior depending on the nature of the aqueous environment and polymer composition. During the swelling process, changes in rheological properties and phase transition properties are observed.

1

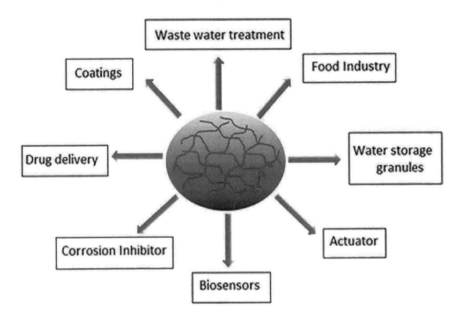

FIGURE 1.1   Applications of hydrogels in various fields.

Hydrogels are also called 'smart gels' because of their sensitivity towards external stimuli like pH, ionic strength, and temperature, which make them highly efficient in various fields like biomedical, sensing, and other industrial applications (Figure 1.1) [4–6].

Generally, hydrogels can be fabricated either by using synthetic or natural polymers. Concerning the biocompatibility, biodegradability, and low cost of natural polymers, hydrogels synthesized from renewable feedstock have been the subject of considerable cognizance during the last few decades. Biopolymer-based hydrogels have been widely used in various fields like hygiene products, agriculture, biomedical materials, heavy metal ions, dyes, biosensors, etc. (Figure 1.2) [7–11]. Several biopolymers such as sodium alginate, starch, hemicelluloses, cellulose, chitin, and their derivatives have been used to develop hydrogels [12–16]. The structures of some of the natural polymers used for the synthesis of hydrogels are given in Figure 1.2.

The virtuous abilities of hydrogels have made them suitable enough for synonyms as smart or intelligent materials, especially in the field of biomedical applications. Their ability to respond under external stimuli like physical/chemical changes and suitable phase transitions with time have focused the research in scaffolds, bioimplants, drug delivery, optics, and others. The physical stimuli include temperature, electric potential, magnetic fields, solvent, light intensity, and pressure. The chemical stimuli include pH, ions, and specific chemical compositions. In most of the cases, the transition in hydrogels on exposure to the external stimuli is reversible. Nature of the monomer, charge density, cross-link density, and the magnitude of external stimuli determine the response of hydrogel [17–19]. In this chapter, we intend to discuss the basics of hydrogels with their properties and applications in various biomedical fields.

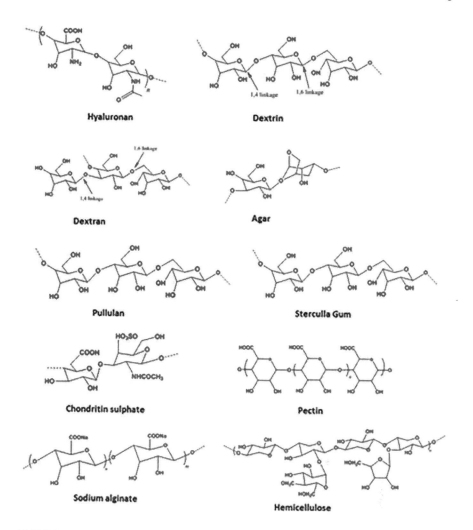

FIGURE 1.2 Chemical structure of different natural polymers.

1.2 HYDROGEL SYNTHESIS

Hydrogels can be synthesized in a number of ways, including single- or multiple-step synthesis processes. The condensation of monomers/ingredients having reactive functional groups with subsequent elimination of side products during the fabrication of polymeric hydrogels mostly follows the basics of polymerization chemistry.

1.2.1 CLASSIFICATION OF HYDROGELS [20]

Hydrogels may be classified depending upon origin, configuration, cross-linking, and application. In the following section, we discuss all the classifications of hydrogels.

1.2.2 CLASSIFICATION BASED ON SOURCE

Hydrogels can be synthesized from polymers with a natural, synthetic, or semi-synthetic origin. Natural polymer-based hydrogels can be prepared from chitosan, sodium alginate, hemicellulose, or cellulose while synthetic hydrogels are mostly synthesized from vinyl monomers using conventional polymerization techniques. The environmental concerns and biomedical requirements, however, led to the focus on natural polymeric hydrogel synthesis over synthetic polymeric hydrogel [21, 22].

1.2.2.1 Based on the Configuration of Polymer Used for Hydrogel Synthesis

Based on their physical and chemical composition, hydrogels can be of the following three types:

- Amorphous: non-crystalline
- Semi-crystalline: A mixture of amorphous and crystalline
- Crystalline

1.2.2.2 According to the Polymeric Composition

According to the composition of the polymer, hydrogels can be classified into three categories: (i) homopolymer hydrogel, (ii) copolymer hydrogel, and (iii) multi-interpenetrating polymeric hydrogel [20].

(i)   Homopolymeric hydrogels are synthesized by using a single species of monomer. The type of monomer and polymerization techniques are key points for the cross-linked structure of homopolymers.

(ii)   Copolymeric hydrogels can be prepared by using two or more kinds of monomeric species in which one of the components is hydrophilic. Copolymerization can lead to different kinds of configurations like random, alternate, or block.

(iii) Interpenetrating polymers are formed using two different polymers and are cross-linked to form a three-dimensional (3D) network structure. In contrast, semi-interpenetrating hydrogels are synthesized having cross-linked polymers as one of the components and a non-cross-linked polymer as the other component.

1.2.2.3 Based on Type of Cross-Linking

Based on the nature of cross-linking, hydrogels can be classified into two categories: chemically cross-linked hydrogels and physically cross-linked hydrogels. The first type of hydrogels are formed via., covalent bonding, resulting in strong cross-linked networks. These are permanent hydrogels and never get dissociated without complete degradation. On the other hand, physically cross-linked hydrogels are formed by secondary forces such as ionic, hydrogen bonding, or hydrophobic interactions. All these physical interactions are reversible and can be disrupted by alterations in physical conditions or application of stress [21].

1.2.3 CLASSIFICATION OVER NETWORK ELECTRICAL CHARGE [23]

Hydrogels can also be classified on the basis of electric charges present on the pendant groups incorporated into the hydrogel backbone. Neutral, cationic, anionic, and amphiphilic hydrogels are with no charges, positive charge, or both negative and positive charges, respectively, on the hydrogel backbone. Examples of neutral, cationic, anionic, and amphiphilic polymers are dextran, carrageenan, chitosan, and collagen, respectively. The presence of different ionic groups along the hydrogel backbone can affect the swelling properties of the hydrogels. Electrostatic interactions between oppositely charged species can form inter- or intramolecular interactions and, hence, consequently affect the different properties of hydrogels.

1.2.4 BASED ON EXTERNAL STIMULI RESPONSE

Another class of hydrogel, which responses to changes in temperature, pH, pressure, irradiation, and chemical stimuli, is called responsive/smart hydrogels. Smart hydrogels undergo fast and reversible changes. The smart polymers can be used for various applications such as biomedical and engineering applications [23].

1.3 METHODS OF HYDROGEL PREPARATION

In general, hydrogels are prepared using hydrophilic polymers or monomers; however, in order to meet the desired properties, hydrophobic monomers have been introduced. Synthetic polymers have good mechanical properties, which results in delayed degradation of the polymeric hydrogel but mostly restrained from in vivo applications. Overall, the main components used to prepare hydrogels are suitable monomers, cross-linkers, and initiators. Various mechanisms for hydrogel preparation are well established in the literature. They can be formulated by various basic techniques like chain-growth polymerization, solution polymerization, suspension polymerization, photo-polymerization, and step-growth polymerization [18, 24].

1.4 APPLICATIONS OF HYDROGELS

Hydrogels have been widely used for different applications because of their water absorption, non-toxicity, and biocompatibility properties. Because of the aforementioned properties, hydrogels have found their way in proteomic, bioseparation, electrophoresis, chromatography, food, diaper, and water remediation applications. Some of the applications of hydrogels are discussed in the next section.

1.4.1 DRUG DELIVERY

The excellent properties of hydrogels make them a great choice in drug delivery applications. Various kinds of drugs can be loaded and released in a controlled manner owing to the porous structure of hydrogels. Further, the sustained release of the drug from the hydrogels can result in the delivery of the active drug to a specific location over a long period of time. The physical and chemical cross-linking can be employed for binding the drug in the hydrogel matrix for sustained release. Different approaches can be employed for enhancing the binding of the loaded drug with that of the hydrogel matrix over a long period of time. The release of the drug can be triggered by both physical and chemical stimuli.

1.4.2 ENVIRONMENTAL APPLICATIONS

Both synthetic and renewable resource-based hydrogels have been used for water remediation applications. Different types of hydrogels prepared from biopolymers have been widely used for heavy metal adsorption. For example, Fe(II), Cu(II), Co(II), Ni(II), Cd(II), As(III), and As(V) are removed from contaminated water using hydrogels prepared from sodium alginate, chitosan, and cellulose.

1.4.3 BIOMEDICAL APPLICATIONS

Hydrogels are attractive candidates for various biomedical applications owing to their unique biocompatibility, chelating nature, and desirable physical and physiological characteristics. Hydrogels serve as carriers for drug and protein entities in a meticulous manner. Water-soluble polymers like poly(acrylic acid), poly(vinyl alcohol), and poly(vinylpyrrolidone) are the most commonly used polymers for hydrogel synthesis. The aforementioned polymers have been used in pharmaceutical and biomedical applications because of their non-toxicity and no requirement of solvent from the system, which eliminates the purification step. The application of hydrogels in biomedical applications includes vaccines, plastic surgery, wound healing, and so on [5, 25, 26].

1.4.4 BIOSENSORS

Biosensors can be prepared by using hydrogels, which act as supports for the immobilization of enzymes. Smart hydrogels are valuable materials for use in biosensors. In the presence of external stimuli, smart hydrogels can help in sensing as well as actuating performance. For instance, the polycarbamoylsulphonate-based hydrogel and others are used for immobilization of the D fructose dehydrogenase enzyme and conducting polymers for sensing application [27, 28].

1.4.5 ADHESIVES

Different kinds of polymeric hydrogels can be used as adhesives because of hydrophobic interactions. In addition, they can be used as sealants for vessels containing corrosive acids.

1.5 CONCLUSION AND FUTURE PERSPECTIVE

Hydrogels are a three-dimensional network of hydrophilic polymers that swell in water while maintaining their basic structure because of chemical or physical cross-linking of individual polymer chains [29, 30]. Hydrogels have many anticipated properties like swelling, mechanical properties, and biocompatible nature which make them suitable in various areas. The swelling properties of hydrogels can be tuned based on the cross-link density. Important applications of hydrogels are in tissue engineering, drug delivery, food and agriculture, industry, and so forth. In addition, hydrogels prepared from natural polymers for use in drug delivery systems are significant as natural polymers are of low cost and are biocompatible and biodegradable in nature. However, the mechanical properties of natural polymer-based hydrogels are not high; hence, we need to modify hydrogels with some monomer/polymer or inorganic nanoparticles which can enhance the mechanical stiffness of the natural polymer-based hydrogels. The future of hydrogels in various applications like sensors, drug delivery, water remediation, and so forth is bright; however, we need to do some collaborative efforts with scientific expertise in different fields in order to commercialize the hydrogels, particularly for use in biomedical applications. More efforts are needed in order to commercialize the hydrogels used in biomedical applications. Innovative methods for the execution of biomaterials in the medical field should be more focused in the future.

1.6 ACKNOWLEDGMENTS

Dr. Shabnam Pathan acknowledges the Department of Science and Technology, Ministry of Science and Technology, India, for the award of fellowship under the Women Scientists Scheme (WOS-B) (ref no. SR/WOS-B/565/2016).

REFERENCES

[1] S. Vasudevan, S. Mohan, G. Sozhan, N.S. Raghavendran, C.V. Murugan, Studies on the oxidation of As (III) to As (V) by in-situ-generated hypochlorite, *Industrial & Engineering Chemistry Research*, 45 (2006) 7729–7732.

[2] O. Wichterle, D. Lim, Hydrophilic gels for biological use, *Nature*, 185 (1960) 117.

[3] D. Das, S. Pal, Modified biopolymer-dextrin based crosslinked hydrogels: application in controlled drug delivery, *RSC Advances*, 5 (2015) 25014–25050.

[4] A. Vashist, A. Vashist, Y. Gupta, S. Ahmad, Recent advances in hydrogel based drug delivery systems for the human body, *Journal of Materials Chemistry B*, 2 (2014) 147–166.

[5] S. Van Vlierberghe, P. Dubruel, E. Schacht, Biopolymer-based hydrogels as scaffolds for tissue engineering applications: a review, *Biomacromolecules*, 12 (2011) 1387–1408.

[6] S. Herrlich, S. Spieth, S. Messner, R. Zengerle, Osmotic micropumps for drug delivery, *Advanced Drug Delivery Reviews*, 64 (2012) 1617–1627.

[7] M. Zohuriaan-Mehr, A. Pourjavadi, H. Salimi, M. Kurdtabar, Protein-and homo poly (amino acid)-based hydrogels with super-swelling properties, *Polymers for Advanced Technologies*, 20 (2009) 655–671.

[8] V. Arbona, D.J. Iglesias, J. Jacas, E. Primo-Millo, M. Talon, A. Gómez-Cadenas, Hydrogel substrate amendment alleviates drought effects on young citrus plants, *Plant and Soil*, 270 (2005) 73–82.

[9] A.R. Kulkarni, K.S. Soppimath, T.M. Aminabhavi, A.M. Dave, M.H. Mehta, Glutaraldehyde crosslinked sodium alginate beads containing liquid pesticide for soil application, *Journal of Controlled Release*, 63 (2000) 97–105.

[10] R-S. Juang, R-C. Shiau, Metal removal from aqueous solutions using chitosan-enhanced membrane filtration, *Journal of Membrane Science*, 165 (2000) 159–167.

[11] F. Abd-Elmohdy, Z. El Sayed, S. Essam, A. Hebeish, Controlling chitosan molecular weight via bio-chitosanolysis, *Carbohydrate Polymers*, 82 (2010) 539–542.

[12] A.W. Chan, R.A. Whitney, R.J. Neufeld, Semisynthesis of a controlled stimuli-responsive alginate hydrogel, *Biomacromolecules*, 10 (2009) 609–616.

[13] C. Elvira, J. Mano, J. San Roman, R. Reis, Starch-based biodegradable hydrogels with potential biomedical applications as drug delivery systems, *Biomaterials*, 23 (2002) 1955–1966.

[14] X-W. Peng, L-X. Zhong, J-L. Ren, R-C. Sun, Highly effective adsorption of heavy metal ions from aqueous solutions by macroporous xylan-rich hemicelluloses-based hydrogel, *Journal of Agricultural and Food Chemistry*, 60 (2012) 3909–3916.

[15] J. Zhou, C. Chang, R. Zhang, L. Zhang, Hydrogels prepared from unsubstituted cellulose in NaOH/urea aqueous solution, *Macromolecular Bioscience*, 7 (2007) 804–809.

[16] X. Shen, J.L. Shamshina, P. Berton, G. Gurau, R.D. Rogers, Hydrogels based on cellulose and chitin: fabrication, properties, and applications, *Green Chemistry*, 18 (2016) 53–75.

[17] M. Bahram, N. Mohseni, M. Moghtader, An introduction to hydrogels and some recent applications, in: *Emerging Concepts in Analysis and Applications of Hydrogels*, IntechOpen, 2016. DOI: 10.5772/64301, location: Head quarters, IntechOpen Limited 7th floor 10 Lower Thames Street London, EC3R 6AF, UK.

[18] A.S. Hoffman, Hydrogels for biomedical applications, *Advanced Drug Delivery Reviews*, 64 (2012) 18–23.

[19] N. Chirani, L. Gritsch, F.L. Motta, S. Fare, History and applications of hydrogels, *Journal of Biomedical Sciences*, 4 (2015).

[20] M.F. Akhtar, M. Hanif, N.M. Ranjha, Methods of synthesis of hydrogels . . . A review, *Saudi Pharmaceutical Journal*, 24 (2016) 554–559.

[21] E.M. Ahmed, Hydrogel: preparation, characterization, and applications: A review, *Journal of Advanced Research*, 6 (2015) 105–121.

[22] A. Ghosal, S. Tiwari, A. Mishra, A. Vashist, N.K. Rawat, S. Ahmad, J. Bhattacharya, Design and engineering of nanogels, in: *Nanogels for Biomedical Applications*, 2017, pp. 9–28 **Book: Nanogels for Biomedical Applications** edited by Arti Vashist, Ajeet K Kaushik, Sharif Ahmad, Madhavan Nair, Pulisher: HYPERLINK "https://books.google.co.in/url?id=i7WrDwAAQBAJ&pg=PA17&q=http://www.rsc.org/shop/books&linkid=1&usg=AFQjCNGY-PZCKTJOQwQKxFyOyjcORUoocw&source=gbs_pub_info_r" Royal Society of Chemistry, CPI group, UK, Ltd.

[23] S. Nesrinne, A. Djamel, Synthesis, characterization and rheological behavior of pH sensitive poly (acrylamide-co-acrylic acid) hydrogels, *Arabian Journal of Chemistry*, 10 (2017) 539–547.

[24] J. Anjali, V.K. Jose, J-M. Lee, Carbon-based hydrogels: synthesis and their recent energy applications, *Journal of Materials Chemistry A*, 7 (2019) 15491–15518.

[25] M.V. Risbud, R.R. Bhonde, Polyacrylamide-chitosan hydrogels: in vitro biocompatibility and sustained antibiotic release studies, *Drug Delivery*, 7 (2000) 69–75.

[26] V.A. Kumar, S. Shi, B.K. Wang, I-C. Li, A.A. Jalan, B. Sarkar, N.C. Wickremasinghe, J.D. Hartgerink, Drug-triggered and cross-linked self-assembling nanofibrous hydrogels, *Journal of the American Chemical Society*, 137 (2015) 4823–4830.

[27] Conducting Polymer Hydrogels: Synthesis, Properties, and Applications for Biosensors, in: *Nanocellulose and Nanohydrogel Matrices*, pp. 175–208. Zhao, Y., Pan, L., Yue, Z. and Shi, Y. (2017), (eds M. Jawaid and F. Mohammad). doi: HYPERLINK "https://doi.org/10.1002/9783527803835.ch8" 10.1002/9783527803835.ch8, John Wiley & Sons, Inc.

[28] Z. Wang, J. Chen, Y. Cong, H. Zhang, T. Xu, L. Nie, J. Fu, Ultrastretchable strain sensors and arrays with high sensitivity and linearity based on super tough conductive hydrogels, *Chemistry of Materials*, 30 (2018) 8062–8069.

[29] A. Vashist, S. Shahabuddin, Y. Gupta, S. Ahmad, Polyol induced interpenetrating networks: chitosan—methylmethacrylate based biocompatible and pH responsive hydrogels for drug delivery system, *Journal of Materials Chemistry B*, 1 (2013) 168–178.

[30] A. Vashist, A. Kaushik, A. Ghosal, J. Bala, R. Nikkhah-Moshaie, W.A. Wani, P. Manickam, M. Nair, Nanocomposite hydrogels: advances in nanofillers used for nanomedicine, *Gels*, 4 (2018) 75.

2 Role of Nanobiotechnology in Hydrogels and Their Medicinal Advancements

Shumaila Shaukat, Yinmao Wei, and Muhammad Arsalan

CONTENTS

2.1 INTRODUCTION TO HYDROGEL

A hydrogel is basically a three-dimensional (3D) network of polymeric chains that can hold huge amount of water (in some cases more than its actual weight) due to physical and chemical cross-linking taking place during the fabrication of structures. The hydrophilic nature of hydrogels is due to presence of -COOH, -SO$_3$H, -NH$_2$, -OH, -CONH$_2$ and -CONH groups. Further, the backbone of hydrogels contains sodium polyacrylate, polyvinyl alcohol, acrylate polymers, and other copolymers with many hydrophilic groups [1]. Sometimes, the cross-linked polymers exist in the form of colloidal gel (water as a dispersion medium). Absorption of water leads to loss of mechanical strength which may cause fracture. The inherent cross-linking and structural coherence prevent crack propagation and maintain the toughness and mechanical properties of hydrogels [2]. In literature the term 'hydrogel' was first used in 1894. Hydrogels were than reported in 1960s by Wichterle and Lim. The natural or synthetic polymeric network of hydrogels shows that they have high absorption capacity (contain 90% water). Material can be termed as a hydrogel only, if atleast 10% of the total weight or volume must be constituted of water. This gives them a higher degree of flexibility similar to natural tissues [3, 4]. Hydrogels undergo gel-sol phase transition in response to physical stimuli like pressure, temperature, magnetic field, electric field, light intensity, solvent composition, or chemical stimuli like ions and pH. The response directly varies with affecting stimulus, and these transitions are reversible at the end of reaction (removal of the trigger) so hydrogels return to their original state [5].

2.2   TECHNICAL FEATURES OF HYDROGELS

Some of the technical or functional features of hydrogel material which make them ideal are listed in the following:

- Hydrogels show highest absorption capacity in saline
- Hydrogels are available at a very cheap cost
- Hydrogels keep the pH neutral after swelling into water
- Hydrogels show highest absorbance capacity under load
- Hydrogels have lowest soluble content and lowest residual monomer
- Hydrogels provide the desired rate of absorption based on requisite of application
- Hydrogels possess high stability and durability during storage
- Following degradation, hydrogels show high biodegradability (no toxic species formed)
- Hydrogels are non-toxic, colorless, and odorless
- Hydrogels show high photostability
- Hydrogels also possess re-wetting capability depending on the applications

2.3   CLASSIFICATION OF HYDROGELS BASED ON DIFFERENT PROPERTIES

A number of classes of hydrogels are reported in the literature. Mainly hydrogels are formed from polyelectrolytes or biopolymers (Figure 2.1). Depending upon the source hydrogels, broadly they have two divisions: synthetic polymers and natural polymers [6]. Based on ionic charges, hydrogels may be anionic, cationic, neutral, or ampholytic. The cross-linking in hydrogels can further be classified into physical gels, chemical gels, and biochemical agents. Similarly, based on structure hydrogels may be crystalline, semi-crystalline, amorphous, or hydrocolloids [7]. Recently hydrogel synthesized from renewable resources has been used in various applications [8, 9].

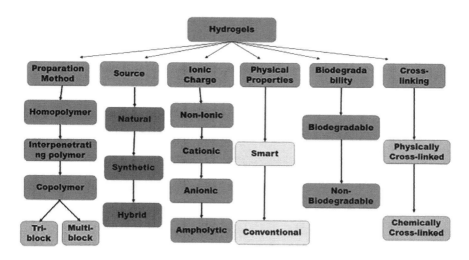

FIGURE 2.1 Classification of hydrogels.

2.4 APPLICATIONS OF HYDROGELS BASED ON SYNTHESIS METHODS

Among the different synthetic hydrogels, largely homopolymer hydrogel (Figure 2.2) consisting of:

Monomer: (i) poly(2-hydroxyethyl methacrylate) (PHEMA), (ii) 2-hydroxy-ethyl methacrylate (HEMA), or (iii) polyethylene glycol (PEG).

Cross-linker: polyethylene glycol dimethacrylate or triethylene glycol dimethacrylate (TEGDMA).

Initiator: benzoin isobutyl ether. They have been largely used in drug delivery systems, scaffolds for protein recombination in tissue engineering, and contact lenses [10, 11].

Hetero or copolymer type hydrogel (Figure 2.3) consisting of methacrylic acid (MMA), polyethylene glycol-polyethylene glycol methacrylate (PEG-PEGMA), carboxymethyl cellulose (CMC), or polyvinylpyrrolidone (PVP) as monomer and triethylene glycol dimethacrylate (TEGDMA) as a cross-linker under free radical photopolymerization. They are mostly used in drug delivery systems and as hydrogel dressing material due to inherent mechanical stability [12, 13]

Hydrogel with a semi-interpenetrating network (Figure 2.4) consisting of acrylamide/acrylic acid copolymer or linear cationic polyallyl ammonium chloride as monomer and N, N'-methylene bisacrylamide as a cross-linker under template copolymerization are used in drug delivery systems [14]. Hydrogel with interpenetrating network consisting of poly(N-isopropyl acrylamide) (PNIPAM) or chitosan as monomer and N, N'-methylene bisacrylamide as a cross-linker in presence of N,N,N',N'-tertramethylethylenediamine (TEMED) and ammonium persulphate (APS) are used in drug delivery systems [15].

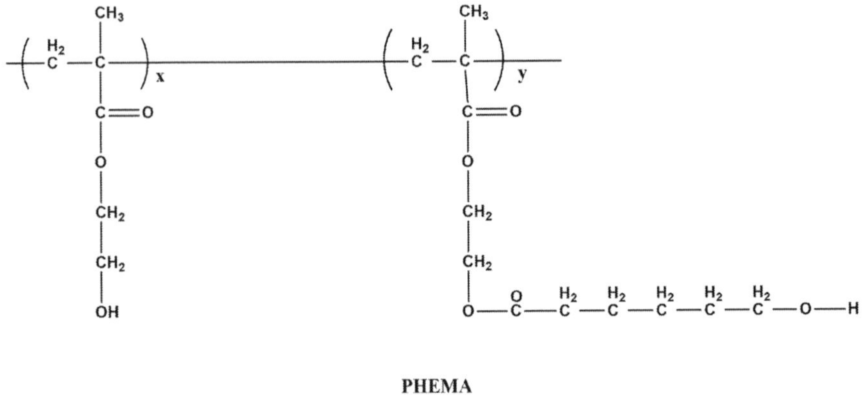

PHEMA

FIGURE 2.2 Structure of homopolymer hydrogel poly(2-hydroxyethyl methacrylate) (PHEMA).

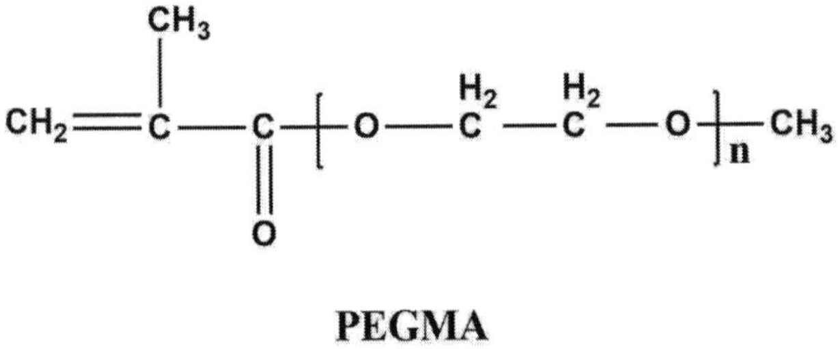

PEGMA

FIGURE 2.3 Structure of polyethylene glycol methacrylate (PEGMA).

Hydrogel with self-assembling peptide systems (Figure 2.5) consisting of acrylate-modified PEG and acrylate-modified hyaluronic acid, heparin or amine end-functionalized 4-arm starPEG as monomer and no cross-linker agent in presence of 1-ethyl-3-(3-dimethylaminopropyl)carbodiimide hydrochloride-N-hydroxy-sulfosuccinimide (EDC/sulfo-NHS) solution at low temperature are used in tissue regeneration [16, 17]. Environmental sensitive hydrogels have the ability to sense pH changes and release their load as a result [13].

2.5 APPLICATION OF HYDROGELS IN DRUG DELIVERY

In drug delivery systems, numerous types of hydrogels are playing a vital role.

2.5.1 pH-Sensitive Hydrogels in Drug Delivery Systems

Structurally pH-sensitive polymers contain acidic or basic group that responds to the environmental pH changes by loss or gain of proton. There are many factors responsible for the hydrogel to be pH sensitive. The use of proper monomer units, with suitable functionalities, interactions, solvents, and response intensities, alters

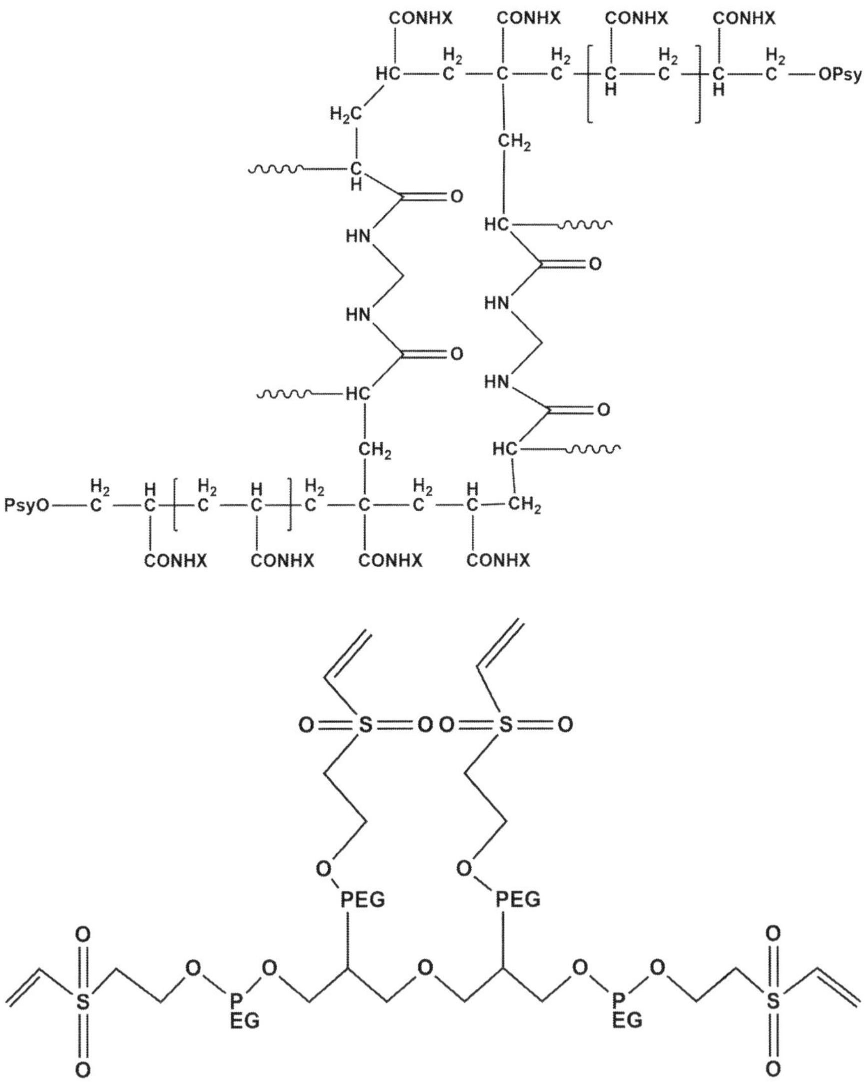

FIGURE 2.4 Structure of (a) Psy-cl-poly(AAm-co-AMPSA) network hydrogel and (b) PEG-based hydrogel.

the kind of drug loading and its release kinetics. The following examples will highlight a few of the important concepts in this regard. Most common of them are polyelectrolytes, which are either anionic or cationic. In basic media, anionic polyelectrolytes like polyacrylic acid (PAA) upon deprotonation allow water molecules to penetrate, causing swelling of hydrogels. However, in acidic media the charge density decreases and the volume collapses. In acidic media, cationic polyelectrolytes like poly (N,N,9-diethylaminoethyl methacrylate) upon ionization allow water molecules to penetrate, causing swelling of hydrogels. Amphiphilic hydrogels exhibit two-phase transitions in basic and acidic media. From collapsed state to expanded

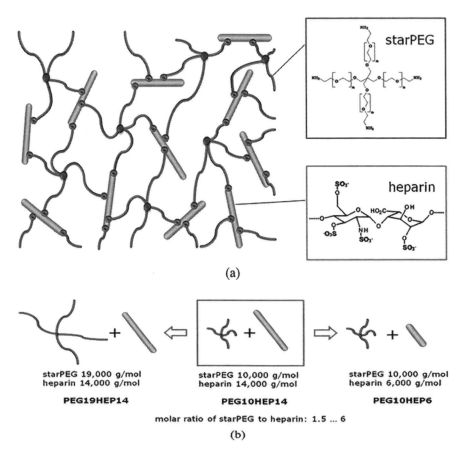

(a)

(b)

FIGURE 2.5   (a) Structure of starPEG heparin hydrogels; (b) variation of heparin and star-PEG building blocks.

Source: Copyright permission © 2011 Petra Birgit Welzel.

state, phase transition occurs in range close to pK_a (dissociation constant) of hydrogel. Hydrogel has two phases: one is a mixed phase, with interactions between solvent and polymer with maximum value of hydrophilicity causing swelling of the hydrogel. The second phase is separated and gel-like, with polymer-polymer interactions with maximum hydrophobicity responsible for shrinkage of the hydrogel. By using different monomers and different pH-sensitive responsive materials, altered degrees of swelling can be achieved. During the study of pH-sensitive hydrogel behavior, most common ionic polymers include poly (acrylamide) (PAA), poly (methyl acrylic acid) (PMAA), poly (dimethylaminoethyl methacrylate) (PDMAEMA), and poly (diethylaminoethyl methacrylate) (PDEAEMA). Phosphoric acid derivative polymers have been also reported as pH-responsive hydrogels [18–20]. For example, the pH-sensitive potential of ES100 (as nanocarrier) for transdermal delivery of a drug (i.e. Piroxicam) has been exploited. They have shown potential to deliver other active drug molecules of BCS class (II and IV) through the transdermal route. Optimized formulation was achieved by using a simple nanoprecipitation technique and response surface quadratic model. Inside the hydrogels, nanoparticles remained stable at acidic pH, and the burst release associated with nanoparticles was reduced. Such systems have shown effective release of drug molecules via in vivo release and ex vivo permeation delivery of nanocarrier in blood circulation. Another example of pH-sensitive hydrogel is 2-hydroxyethyl acrylate (2-HEA) grafted carboxymethyl chitosan (CmCHT), which has shown potential application in controlled transdermal drug delivery systems [21, 22]. Hybrid hydrogels with semi-interpenetrating polymer networks, containing self-assembled collagen nanofibrils as pH-sensitive components, have been used for controlled release of methyl violet as a model drug. Content of PNIPAM had great effect on the drug release abilities of the hydrogel. Semi-IPNs possess different swelling behavior under different pH, making them sensitive collagen-based hybrid hydrogels with great importance in controlled drug delivery systems [23]. The pH-sensitive hydrogel composed of poly (methacrylic acid) (PMAA) grafted with polyethylene glycol (PEG) is also reported for controlled drug delivery of salmon calcitonin (an oral drug). In vitro studies revealed that salmon calcitonin was successfully incorporated and released from the system due to variation in pH level. There is ionic interaction between polymer and hydrogel whereas the solvent used in the hydrogel affects the loading efficiency of the system. The transport mechanism is found suitable for oral drug delivery of peptides [24]. A hydrophilic hybrid pH-sensitive hydrogel system composed of poly (methacrylic acid) (PMAA) grafted with polyethylene glycol (PEG) and acryloyl group modified cholesterol bearing pullulan (CHPOA) nanogel has been developed for controlled delivery of pregabalin (an anticonvulsant drug). By altering hydrophobicities and cross-linking agents, this system could be used for stimuli-responsive drug delivery (Figure 2.6) [25].

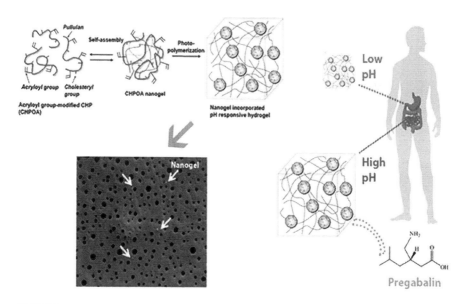

FIGURE 2.6 pH-sensitive hydrogel system for the controlled delivery of pregabalin (PGB).

Source: Copyright permission © 2017 Gunce E. Cinay.

For colon-specific drugs, release development of two azo hydrogels containing acryloyl chloride modified olsalazine copolymerized with hydroxyethyl methacrylate and methacrylic acid for pH-responsive release has been reported. This system is a novel chemotherapeutic strategy for treatment of colon cancer. Moreover, pH-specific interpolymeric hydrogels based on chitosan and polyvinyl alcohol with glutaraldehyde are utilized for the release of naproxen in colon targeted drug delivery. Another pH-sensitive semi-IPN hydrogel based on poly (aspartic acid) and starch with potential applicability for colon-specific drug delivery system has been reported as a potential oral drug delivery system. The release of 5-Fluorouracil has been studied with and without enzyme (α-amylase) simulated gastrointestinal conditions. A novel biodegradable hydrogel Dextran methacrylate succinic acid (Dex-MA-SA) and poly (N-2-hydroxyethyl)-DL aspartamide (PHEA) have been synthesized for colon specific drug (Model drug: 2-methoxyestradiol) delivery system (PHM-SA). The enzymatic degradability along with mucoadhesion and cell compatibility of Dex-MA-SA and PHEA hydrogel systems are useful for oral treatment of colonic cancer. An optimized oral delivered Zein-co-acrylic acid hydrogel incorporated with rutin (Ru) and 5-florouracil (5-Fu) has been reported for less toxic anticancer activity (Figure 2.7). These hybrid hydrogels are a favorable vector for anticancer drugs against breast cancer and for oral drug delivery [26–30]. The pH-sensitive hydrogels based on cellulose nanofibers and polyvinyl alcohol are suitable for controlled released drug delivery systems for cisplatin anticancer drugs of the small intestine [31]. The pH-sensitive CPCS hydrogels based on pachyman and its carboxymethylated (CMP) also highlighted the usefulness in controlled oral drug release of bovine serum albumin [32].

2.5.2 TEMPERATURE-SENSITIVE HYDROGELS IN DRUG DELIVERY SYSTEMS

Similar to pH responsiveness, temperature-sensitive hydrogels are also greatly favored due to their uniqueness and possible applications in biomedical applications (Figure 2.8). Hybrid hydrogels with semi-interpenetrating polymer networks, containing poly (N-iso-propylacrylamide) (PNIPAM) as thermo-sensitive components, are used for controlled release of methyl violet as a model drug. As compared to native collagen, semi-IPNs showed better elastic properties and thermal stability. Semi-IPNs possess different swelling behavior under different temperatures. Content of PNIPAM had a great effect on drug release abilities and temperature sensitivity. The drug release behavior in vitro for semi-IPNs revealed tunable performance for release ability. So, the thermo-responsive mechanism of semi-IPNs for sensitive collagen-based hybrid hydrogels revealed their great importance in controlled drug delivery systems [23]. Dual thermo- and pH-responsive hydrogels loaded with doxorubicin (DOX) have potential dual therapy against breast cancer. The accelerated release of doxorubicin in lower concentrations was confirmed to be the trigger for effective anticancer ability. Hydrogels are cytocompatible, and their potential for local therapy of breast cancer is demonstrated by the proliferation of MCF-7 cells on DOX-loaded hydrogels evaluated by 4',6-diamidino-2-phenylindole staining [33].

A dual thermo- and pH-sensitive system holds better prospects and control over the drug delivery process. The idea is to identify the pH-sensitive moieties followed by suitable modification to make them thermo-sensitive materials. A chitosan-poly

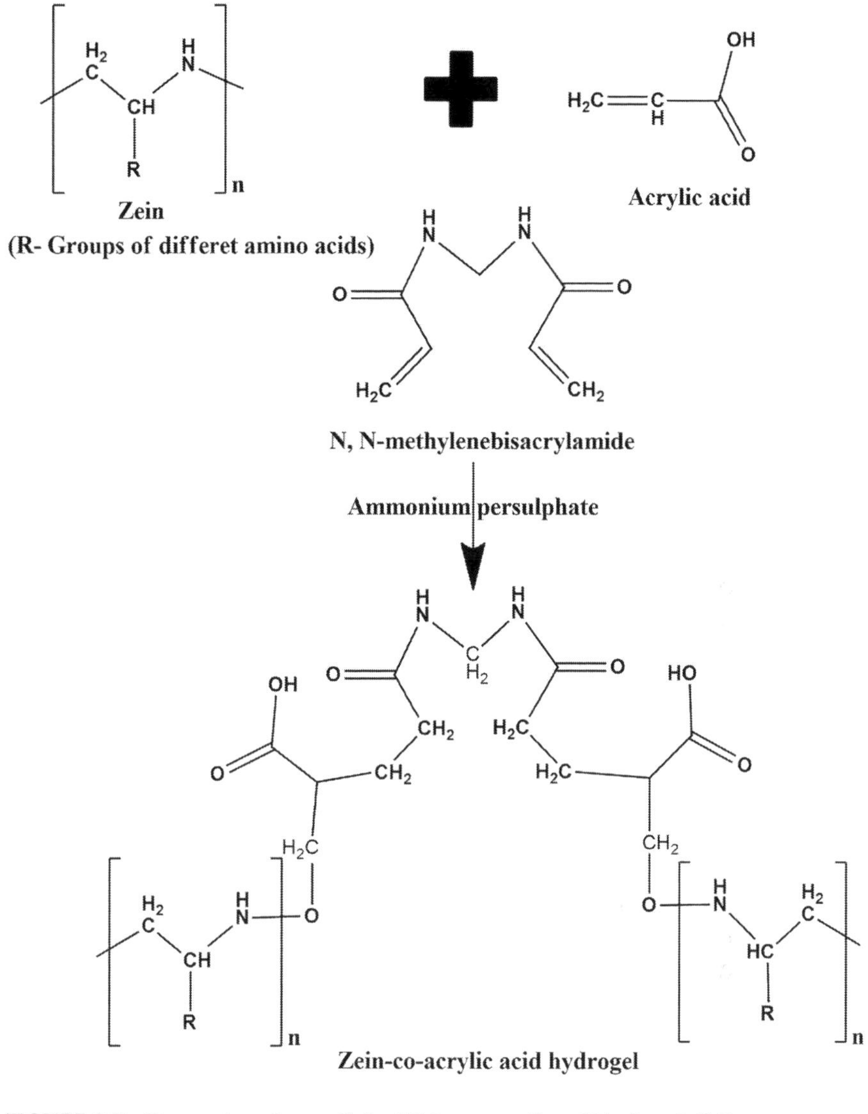

FIGURE 2.7   Preparation of cross-linked Zein-co-acrylic acid hydrogel. [35]

(ethylene oxide) semi-interpenetrating polymer network is developed as a pH-sensitive hydrogel for pH-dependent and localized drug delivery in the stomach. At low pH, chitosan-PEO semi-IPN swell extensively in simulated gastric fluid (SGF) due to ionization of glucosamine residues [34]. A new pH-sensitive hydrogel synthesized via graft copolymerization between salecan and 2-acrylamido-2-methyl-1-propanesulfonic acid is used for controlled drug delivery of insulin [35]. Dual thermo- and pH-sensitive grafted hydrogel poly (N,N-dimethylaminoethyl methacrylate-co-propargyl acrylate) P (DMAEMA-co-ProA) have been developed

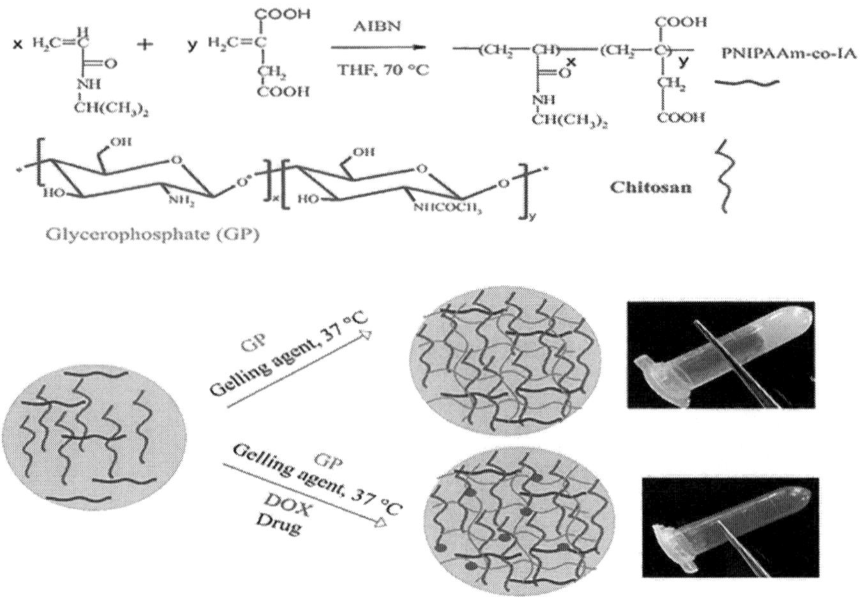

FIGURE 2.8   Schematic representation of hydrogel preparation.

Source: Copyright permission © 2019 Marziyeh Fathi.

subsequently due to dual stimulus-response exhibiting fast response and high swelling ratio. The release rate of drug molecules can be modulated by pH and temperature [36]. Temperature-sensitive hydrogel-based molecularly imprinted polymers (hydro MIPs) are obtained via frontal polymerization. In vivo evaluation show that hydro MIPs showed higher bioavailability [37]. Poly (amino ester urethane) (PAEU) copolymers are reported as potential hydrogels for drug delivery because of their non-toxicity and ability to exhibit sol-gel phase transition with increasing temperature. This copolymer is cytocompatible as a viable hydrogel system for controlled release of the anticancer drug doxorubicin (DOX). Moreover, the potential application to chemoembolization in liver cancer treatment is also confirmed. A novel chitosan/hyaluronic acid/β-sodium glycerophosphate (CS/HA/GP) hydrogel system demonstrates adhesion to cancer cells. The doxorubicin drug-loaded hydrogel solution is transformed to gel upon increase of body temperature. Moreover, CS/HA/GP hydrogels show good affinity to cancer cells, indicating potential application in tumor site–specific release of drugs [38, 39]. Xylan-based P (NIPAm-co-AA) temperature-sensitive hydrogel had excellent swelling kinetic abilities (Figure 2.9). Therefore, it has a unique application as a vector for intestinal targeted oral acetylsalicylic acid drug delivery carrier [40].

Thermo-sensitive hydrogels loaded with silver nanoparticles (HG-AgNPs) are versatile, cost-effective with adequate gelation time, and optimal for in situ biomedical applications. HG-AgNPs shorten surgery time and reduce risk of infection as they possess antimicrobial antibiotic-free property [41]. Temperature-sensitive poly

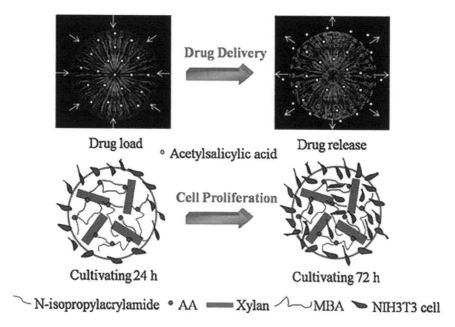

FIGURE 2.9 Diagram of drug delivery behaviors and cell proliferation of the xylan-based P(NIPAm-g-AA) hydrogels.

Source: Copyright permission © 2016 Cundian Gao.

(NIPAAm-co-AAc) hydrogel is loaded with riboflavin (vitamin B2), which releases drugs with increase in temperature. Artificial neural networks and MATLAB were used to model the release data [42].

2.6 APPLICATION OF HYDROGELS FROM NANOTECHNOLOGICAL PERSPECTIVE

Nowadays, nanotechnology has further enhanced the utility of hydrogels in the medicinal field. In the emerging world, hydrogels are also finding applications in dyes and heavy metal ions removal, water purification, scaffolds in tissue engineering, contact lenses, biosensors, regeneration purposes, cell-based therapies, carriers in controlled drug delivery systems, therapies, and immune isolation systems, etc. Mostly the nanotechnology has led to in situ generations of nanoplatforms within the hydrogel systems or nanocomposite hydrogel systems where already prepared nanoparticles are incorporated in the hydrogel system. In both situations the nanoentities are known to improve the mechanical strength of the overall system and alter the physical or chemical stability of the material. Functionalized nanoentities work as vertices or cores for improvement in the cross-linking efficiency and channelize few biochemical reactions. Some of the applications of hydrogels that are greatly improved by nanotechnology are discussed here.

2.6.1   APPLICATION OF HYDROGELS IN DYE REMOVAL

Mesoporous lignocellulose hydrogel materials containing lignin, cellulose, and hemicellulose with enhanced mechanical properties are prepared by the formation of Si-O-C cross-links among lignocellulosic fibrils. The addition of APTES as a silane-based coupling agent increases dynamic storage modulus as compared to unmodified gel. The prepared gel includes the interesting properties of weathering and dye adsorption [43]. A new bio-based organic-inorganic hybrid nanocomposite hydrogel named cellulose nanowhisker-graft-polymerized acrylic acid/layer double hydroxide (cellulose nanowhisker-graft-PAA/LDH) has been developed to enhance dye removal efficiency. The removal efficiency remained stable up to three cycles, which proves cellulose nanowhisker-graft-PAA/LDH hydrogel to be a potential adsorbent for water treatment [44]. A biocompatible glycidyl methacrylate substituted dextran with poly acrylic acid (Dex-MA-PAA) hydrogel adsorbent for the removal of cationic dyes from aqueous solution. The dye removal efficiency for crystal violet and methylene blue reached 86.4% and 93.9% respectively within one minute. The removal efficiency remained >95% after five cycles, which proves Dex-MA-PAA hydrogel as an efficient adsorbent in water treatment. Another environmentally friendly hydrogel, TiO_2-Gum-Tragacanth (TGTH), has adsorption capacity for removal of methylene blue from simulated-color solution. The cationic dye removal process was a modeled radial basis function neural network (RBFNN); results propose TGTH as a proper adsorbent for the dye removal process [45, 46]. A novel poly (acrylic acid) (PAA)-based super-adsorbent nanocomposite hydrogel (NC gel) has been prepared via free radical in situ polymerization. Due to the exposure of a large number of active sites, the adsorption capacity for methylene blue (MB) is as high as 2,100 mg/g near-neutral pH. Such high adsorption capacity was noted for the first time towards removal of MB. PAA-based super-adsorbent NC gel is of great application in removal of organic/cationic dyes from industrial effluents, and by choosing optimal nanospherulites (CNSs) as a cross-linker, it should be applicable for removal of dye pollution [47]. A magnetic poly (aspartic acid)-poly (acrylic acid) hydrogel (PAsp-PAA/Fe_3O_4) with semi-interpenetrating network showing maximum adsorption capacity toward organic dye methylene blue and neutral red (NR) has been prepared. The hydrogel possesses good reproducibility, high swelling ratio, pH sensitivity, and excellent adsorption for dye pollutant removal from wastewater [48]. The lignin-based hydroxyethyl cellulose-PVA (LCP) super-absorbent hydrogel with high swelling ratio, good water retention, and biodegradability could take up a large amount of positively charged dyes including rhodamine 6G, MB, and crystal violet (Figure 2.10). LCP hydrogels are of great application in the fields of commercial diapers, soil-water retention, dye removal, and seed cultivation [49].

Many novel magnetic hydrogels with high water absorbance, such as AAm/AMPS hydrogel, AAm/AMPS/PEG semi-IPNs, Mag-AAm/AMPS/PEG semi-IPNs, and Mag-AAm/AMPS hydrogel, have been synthesized. Janus Green B model proves these hydrogels as of great application in wastewater treatment and dye uptake [50].

2.6.2   APPLICATION OF HYDROGELS IN HEAVY METAL IONS REMOVAL

Polyacrylic acid diallyl dimethyl ammonium chloride (AAC-Dadmac) hydrogel is used for the removal of heavy metals like copper(II), nickel(II), zinc(II), and chromium.

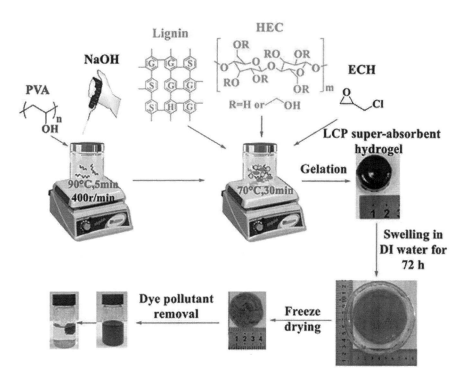

FIGURE 2.10 Preparation scheme and application of LCP super-absorbent hydrogel.

Source: Copyright permission © 2019 Siqi Huang.

The results proved AAC-Dadmac hydrogel to be a good adsorbent for removal of heavy metal ions from electroplating wastewater [51]. A novel MnO_2 nanotubes@ reduced graphene oxide hydrogel (MNGH) has been synthesized via one-step hydrothermal co-assembly. MNGH shows adsorption capacity towards many heavy metal ions such as Pb^{2+}, Cd^{2+}, Ag^+, Zn^{2+}, and Cu^{2+} after multiple adsorption-desorption cycles. Thus, MNGH serves as a potential adsorbent for the efficient removal of heavy metal ions from wastewater [52]. Similarly, Chitosan/gelatin spherical (CG) hydrogel particles were fabricated by inverse emulsion for the removal of co-existing heavy metal ions like Hg(II), Pb(II), Cd(II) and Cr(III) from natural and industrial wastes (Figure 2.11). [53].

A new kind of hydrogel with excellent mechanical properties, low cost, and high efficiency for Cu^{2+} removal has been synthesized and named as carboxymethyl chitosan-kaolinite composite hydrogel (CMCS-Kaolin composite hydrogel). Composite hydrogels are easily regenerated and reused and hence are used as effective adsorbents for removal of heavy metal ions [54]. A natural sodium alginate/polyethyleneimine (ALG/PEI) composite hydrogel is also effective for treatment and recycling of heavy metal ions in wastewater [55]. Super-absorbent polymer hydrogel (SPH) prepared via free radical polymerization is reported for efficient removal of Ni^{2+}, Cd^{2+}, Co^{2+}, and Cu^{2+} from aqueous solution at pH 2–10 [56]. At neutral pH gelatin-chitosan

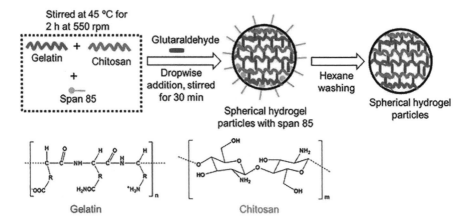

FIGURE 2.11   Preparation of CG hydrogel particles for heavy metal ion adsorption.

Source: Copyright permission © 2019 Suguna Perumal.

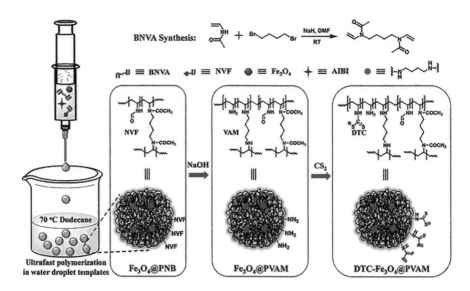

FIGURE 2.12   Fabrication of DTC-Fe$_3$O$_4$@PVAM hydrogel beads.

Source: Copyright permission © 2019 Xin Wang.

hydrogel particles are used to remove heavy metal ions such as Hg(II), Cd(II), Pb(II), and Cr(III) from wastewater [57]. Size controlled millimeter-scale hydrogel beads named as dithiocarbamate-decorated poly(vinyl amine) (DTC-Fe$_3$O$_4$@PVAM) hydrogel beads (Figure 2.12) with good adsorption capacity have been synthesized for water environment remediation [58].

2.6.3 HYDROGELS AS SCAFFOLDS IN TISSUE ENGINEERING

As scaffolds, hydrogels play role in tissue repairing (bone, cartilage, spinal cord, artificial muscle, and nerve regeneration) in tissue engineering. Biomolecules are processed into scaffold and hydrogel systems in situ during the formation of hydrogels and thus used in tissue engineering applications for controlled delivery of cells-specific biomolecules [59]. Hydrogel scaffolds by variation of stiffness using digital light processing-based 3D printing play an important role in tissue engineering (bone and cartilage regeneration). Constructing a cell-seedling hydrogel with different stiffness is useful for muscle and cartilage regeneration [60, 61]. Incorporation of magneto-electric material into hydrogel-based scaffolds results in the formation of $CoFe_2O_4$/methacrylated gellan gum (GGMA) poly(vinylidene fluoride) (PVDF) hydrogel-based scaffold, which is applicable in bone tissue engineering [62]. Hydrogel scaffold of silk fibroin/oxidized pectin (SF/OP) is loaded with Vanco HCl to prevent bone infection [63]. Eggshell microparticle (ESP) reinforced hydrogel is suitable for bone, tooth, tendon, and cartilage repair and bone regeneration applications, as it can easily be incorporated into 3D scaffolds. ESP-reinforced scaffolds are of application in dental, cranial, and maxillofacial aspects [64]. The two glycosaminoglycan are incorporated into silylated hydroxypropylmethylcellulose-based hydrogel (Si-HPMC) to build a scaffold for bone and cartilage tissue engineering as it possesses highest compressive modulus [65]. A new approach of developing collagen/fibrin hydrogel (Figure 2.13) as a matrix for stem cells results in better cell proliferation and provides a 3D microenvironment for bone tissue regeneration [66].

Osseo-integration is essential for bone regeneration; due to this, osteoconductive hydrogel Hydroxyapatite mineralized polyacrylamide urethacrylate dextran (Hap-PADH) hydrogel has been synthesized. This improves adhesion, proliferation, and osteoconductivity for bone repairing [67]. Nanocellulose, along with sodium alginate, is

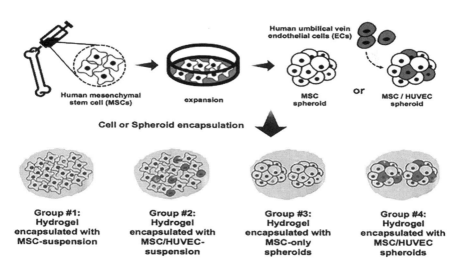

FIGURE 2.13 Process to fabricate collagen/fibrin hydrogel.

Source: Copyright permission © 2019 Dong Nyoung Heo.

used to 3D print hydrogels for cartilage engineering with good regeneration. Application of vitreous humor (VH) as an ECM hydrogel results in no proliferation and is a source to fabricate cartilaginous hydrogel for tissue engineering. In cartilage tissue engineering (CTE), the extrusion-based bioprinting (EBB) technique is the most progressive (Figure 2.14). The bio-inks in CTE should be biocompatible, printable, and mechanically good. By using hydrogel or self-supporting hydrogel, bioprinting fabrication of chondral, osteochondral, and cartilage for regeneration is done [68–70].

Hyaluronic acid hydrogel with ligament stem cells (human periodontal ligament stem cells (hPLSCs)) for cartilage tissue engineering has been reported with improved biocompatibility, porous interconnected structure, more stiffness and longer retention time of stem cells [67, 71]. For the treatment of damaged spinal cord tissues, hydrogel loaded with neurotrophin-3(NT-3) factor results in increased recovery. The hydrogel+NT-3 reduces the collagen deposit and glial scarring, resulting in regeneration of neuronal tissues. Thus, it is an effective growth factor and biomaterial-based therapy for spinal cord injury [72]. Hydrogel scaffold based on hyaluronic acid and peptide PPFLMLLKGSTR function in synergy to strengthen and restore injured spinal cords. Cellular survival and adhesive growth of stem cells are improved using a hyaluronic acid–based scaffold [73]. A new hydrogel microfiber scaffold with cross-linking of gelatin methacryloyl has been developed for regeneration of injured spinal cords. GeIMA hydrogel possesses lower Young's modulus and soaks more water and promotes angiogenesis and, thus, is suitable for neuronal cells [74]. The swelling, conductive, and mechanical properties of electro-responsive grepheneoxide-poly(acrylic acid) hydrogel makes it compatible with bone marrow–derived stem cells and, thus, is used in artificial muscle and tissue engineering scaffolds [75]. Two sets of

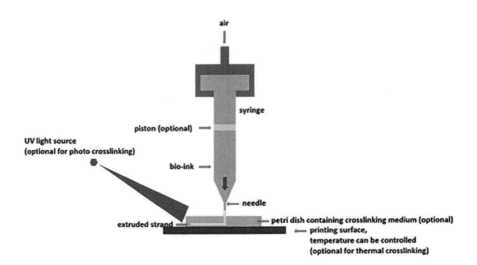

FIGURE 2.14   Schematic of extrusion-based bioprinting using various cross-linking mechanisms.

Source: Copyright permission © 2017 Fu You.

poly(amidoamine) hydrogel as scaffold obtained by polyaddition of piperazine with N,N'-methylenebis(acrylamide) are utilized for in vivo nerve regeneration [76].

2.6.4 HYDROGELS FOR CONTACT LENSES

Commercial hydrogel contact lenses via ocular delivery are used in the treatment of glaucoma. Vitamin E integrated polymeric hydrogel is useful for feasible delivery of prostaglandin and effective for glaucoma management. Moreover, glaucoma therapy is effective by bimatoprost eluting contact lenses [77]. Due to increased hydrophobicity, silicon hydrogels are of potential application in drug delivery from contact lenses. PEG containing silicon hydrogels are important for antibiotic delivery. TRIS-co-PEG silicon with high transparency, good refractive index, wettability, and protein repulsion can influence the drug release [78]. Silicon-based hydrogel contact lenses with high oxygen permeability, stiffness, protein adsorption, and hydrophilicity with non-cytotoxicity hence are feasible for making contact lenses [79].

2.7 ROLE OF DNA HYDROGEL INTEGRATED NANOCHANNELS

Among responsive molecules existing in nanochannels, DNA hydrogels are a three-dimensional network which provides the gating mechanism of a single nanochannel (Figure 2.15). DNA hydrogels possess high ion flux, high rectification ratio, and

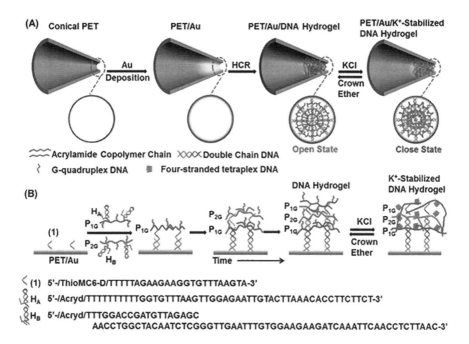

FIGURE 2.15 Preparation process of the ion channel.

Source: Copyright permission © 2018 Yafeng Wu.

multiple gating features. Thus, they are applicable to sensors, microfluidic systems, and desalination devices [80]. DNA/poly(lactic-co-glycolic acid) (DNA/PLGA) hybrid hydrogels (HDNA) with porous structure are used in water-insoluble ophthalmic therapeutic delivery. Dexamethasone (DEX) was used as model system. An HDNA-based delivery system possesses unique treatment paradigms and is applicable for treatment of various eye diseases [81]. A new Lamb-Wave based device has been introduced for detection of DNA amplification via rolling circle amplification (RCA). The formation of DNA hydrogel during RCA is monitored by increase of viscosity at 30°C and applied voltage of 17V. This lab-on-a-chip-based device provides simple and low-cost diagnosis of infectious diseases and is applicable to clinical settings [82]. A new target-responsive DNA hydrogel has been used to construct biosensors for adenosine detection in urine. In order to prepare DNA hydrogel acrydite modified single strand DNA, acrydite modified single strand adenosine aptamer and hemin aptamer are used. Au@HKUST-1 is coated with DNA hydrogel. In the presence of hemin, hydrogel remains in a gel state, forming G-quadruplex/hemin with removal of excess hemin. The addition of adenosine results in complete dissolution of DNA hydrogel and release of G-quadruplex/hemin and Au@HKUST-1, resulting in strong "signal on" readout and, thus, a novel biosensor in the field of biotechnology [83]. A pattern-formation-based system, DNA logic gate immobilized in gel for biological morphologies has been synthesized, thus resulting in a Voroni pattern in two-dimensional hydrogel medium to control solidification and solubilization of gels by DNA. This structured gel is of use in sustained drug release and artificial organ formation [84]. A DNA hydrogel amplified platform for detection of miRNA has been developed with dyes and quantum dots to assemble signal probes. DNA hydrogel works as a fluorescence signal amplifier for miRNA-141 detection over very wide linear detection ranges. This method is applicable to miRNA-141 detection in human prostate cancer with good sensing strategy and biomedical analysis [85].

2.8   CONCLUSIONS

This chapter aims to introduce hydrogels, technical features of hydrogels, and classification of hydrogels based on different physical and chemical properties. On the basis of these properties, there are numerous applications of hydrogels by modifying their basic structure. Among the numerous applications of hydrogels, their uses in controlled drug delivery, tissue engineering, contact lenses, and a few others are discussed here.

2.9   FUTURE PERSPECTIVE

Focus on in vivo studies of pH-sensitive ES100 nanocarrier in order to establish its potential use for transdermal delivery of drugs. Manner of action recommends collagen/PNIPAM/semi-IPNs as biomaterial in pharmaceutical fields and tissue engineering applications as carrier matrices. In order to control the delivery rate of polypeptides for oral drug delivery, the amount of diluent should be controlled specifically in case of salmon calcitonin. The pH-sensitive hydrogel consisting of P (MAA-g-EG) and acryloyl group modified cholesterol bearing pullulan (CHPOA) nanogel could be applicable in clinical aspects for pH-trigger release of therapeutic molecules. Azo hydrogels could be potential carriers for colon-specific drug delivery. The pH-responsive hydrogel-based on chitosan holds great promise to be applied as a carrier in anticancer drug delivery. Salecan grafted 2-acrylamido-2-methyl-1-propanesulfonic acid hydrogel can be of great importance for controlled oral drug delivery, especially for protein/peptide therapeutics. A semi-IPN hydrogel based on poly (aspartic acid) and starch due to excellent pH-sensitive release property could be used for oral treatment of colonic cancer via drug delivery systems. CPCS hydrogels based on pachyman and its carboxymethylated (CMP) opens a new space for pachyman developing, which would be of great application in biochemical and pharmaceutical fields. The extrusion-based bioprinting (EBB) technique for cartilage reconstruct for living implants is of important interest in future clinical applications. In future the hyaluronic acid-based scaffold used for spinal cord regeneration can be enhanced by gene transfection and useful for neural stem cell implantation. DNA hydrogel-based sensors for the online detection of targets can be built in future researches (e.g. adenosine detection).

REFERENCES

[1] V. K. Thakur and M. R. Kessler, "Self-healing polymer nanocomposite materials: A review," *Polymer (Guildf)*, vol. 69, pp. 369–383, 2015.

[2] D. S. Warren, S. P. H. Sutherland, J. Y. Kao, G. R. Weal, and S. M. Mackay, "The preparation and simple analysis of a clay nanoparticle composite hydrogel," *J. Chem. Educ.*, vol. 94, no. 11, pp. 1772–1779, 2017.

[3] V. K. Thakur and M. K. Thakur, "Recent advances in graft copolymerization and applications of chitosan: A review," *ACS Sustain. Chem. Eng.*, vol. 2, no. 12, pp. 2637–2652, 2014.

[4] V. K. Thakur and M. K. Thakur, "Recent trends in hydrogels based on psyllium polysaccharide: A review," *J. Clean. Prod.*, vol. 82, pp. 1–15, 2014.

[5] O. Wichterle, and D. Lim, "Hydrophilic gels for biological use." *Nature*, vol, 185, pp.117–118, 1960.

[6] M. Bessodes, A. K. A. Silva, D. Scherman, O-W. Merten, and C. Richard, "Growth Factor Delivery Approaches in Hydrogels," *Biomacromolecules*, vol. 10, no. 1, pp. 9–18, 2008.

[7] F. Ullah, M. B. H. Othman, F. Javed, Z. Ahmad, and H. M. Akil, "Classification, processing and application of hydrogels: A review," *Mater. Sci. Eng. C.*, vol. 57, pp. 414–433, 2015.

[8] H. D. Sparks *et al.*, "Flowable Polyethylene Glycol Hydrogels Support the in Vitro Survival and Proliferation of Dermal Progenitor Cells in a Mechanically Dependent Manner," *ACS Biomater. Sci. Eng.*, vol. 5, no. 2, pp. 950–958, 2019.

[9] N. Das, "Preparation methods and properties of hydrogel: A review," *Int. J. Pharm. Pharm. Sci.*, vol. 5, no. 3, pp. 112–117, 2013.

[10] B. Kim and N. A. Peppas, "Poly(ethylene glycol)-containing hydrogels for oral protein delivery applications," *Biomed. Microdevices*, vol. 5, no. 4, pp. 333–341, 2003.

[11] A. Cretu, R. Gattin, L. Brachais, and D. Barbier-Baudry, "Synthesis and degradation of poly (2-hydroxyethyl methacrylate)-graft-poly (ε-caprolactone) copolymers," *Polym. Degrad. Stab.*, vol. 83, no. 3, pp. 399–404, 2004.

[12] Y. Zhang, F. Wu, M. Li, and E. Wang, "PH switching on-off semi-IPN hydrogel based on cross-linked poly(acrylamide-co-acrylic acid) and linear polyallyamine," *Polymer (Guildf)*, vol. 46, no. 18, pp. 7695–7700, 2005.

[13] A. Richter, G. Paschew, S. Klatt, J. Lienig, K. Arndt, and H. P. Adler, "<Sensors-08–00561. Pdf>," vol. c, pp. 561–581, 2008.

[14] C. Alvarez-Lorenzo, A. Concheiro, A. S. Dubovik, N. V. Grinberg, T. V. Burova, and V. Y. Grinberg, "Temperature-sensitive chitosan-poly(N-isopropylacrylamide) interpenetrated networks with enhanced loading capacity and controlled release properties," *J. Control. Release*, vol. 102, no. 3, pp. 629–641, 2005.

[15] D. Macaya and M. Spector, "Injectable hydrogel materials for spinal cord regeneration: A review," *Biomed. Mater.*, vol. 7, no. 1, 2012.

[16] Y. Brudno and D. J. Mooney, "On-demand drug delivery from local depots," *J. Control. Release*, vol. 219, pp. 8–17, 2015.

[17] P. B. Welzel *et al.*, "Modulating biofunctional starPEG heparin hydrogels by varying size and ratio of the constituents," *Polymers (Basel)*, vol. 3, no. 1, pp. 602–620, 2011.

[18] A. K. Bajpai, J. Bajpai, R. Saini, and R. Gupta, "Responsive polymers in biology and technology," *Polym. Rev.*, vol. 51, no. 1, pp. 53–97, 2011.

[19] K. Na, K. H. Lee, and Y. H. Bae, "pH-sensitivity and pH-dependent interior structural change of self-assembled hydrogel nanoparticles of pullulan acetate/oligo-sulfonamide conjugate," *J. Control. Release*, vol. 97, no. 3, pp. 513–525, 2004.

[20] M. Qindeel, N. Ahmed, F. Sabir, S. Khan, and A. Ur-Rehman, "Development of novel pH-sensitive nanoparticles loaded hydrogel for transdermal drug delivery," *Drug Dev. Ind. Pharm.*, vol. 45, no. 4, pp. 629–641, 2019.

[21] H. J. Jeong, S. J. Nam, J. Y. Song, and S. N. Park, "Synthesis and physicochemical properties of pH-sensitive hydrogel based on carboxymethyl chitosan/2-hydroxyethyl acrylate for transdermal delivery of nobiletin," *J. Drug Deliv. Sci. Technol.*, vol. 51, no. October 2018, pp. 194–203, 2019.

[22] C. Ding, M. Zhang, M. Ma, J. Zheng, Q. Yang, and R. Feng, "Thermal and pH dual-responsive hydrogels based on semi-interpenetrating network of poly(N-isopropylacrylamide) and collagen nanofibrils," *Polym. Int.*, no. April, 2019.

[23] M. Torres-Lugo and N. A. Peppas, "Molecular design and in vitro studies of novel pH-sensitive hydrogels for the oral delivery of calcitonin," *Macromolecules*, vol. 32, no. 20, pp. 6646–6651, 1999.

[24] G. E. Cinay *et al.*, "Nanogel-integrated pH-responsive composite hydrogels for controlled drug delivery," *ACS Biomater. Sci. Eng.*, vol. 3, no. 3, pp. 370–380, 2017.

[25] Z. Ma, R. Ma, X. Wang, J. Gao, Y. Zheng, and Z. Sun, "Enzyme and PH responsive 5-flurouracil (5-FU)loaded hydrogels based on olsalazine derivatives for colon-specific drug delivery," *Eur. Polym. J.*, vol. 118, no. May, pp. 64–70, 2019.

[26] N. González-Vidal, A. Martínez De Ilarduya, and S. Muñoz-Guerra, "Poly(ethylene-co-1,4-cyclohexylenedimethylene terephthalate) copolyesters obtained by ring opening polymerization," *J. Polym. Sci. Part A—Polym. Chem.*, vol. 47, no. 22, pp. 5954–5966, 2009.

[27] C. Liu, X. Gan, and Y. Chen, "A novel pH-sensitive hydrogels for potential colon-specific drug delivery: Characterization and in vitro release studies," *Starch/Staerke*, vol. 63, no. 8, pp. 503–511, 2011.

[28] F. F. Azhar, E. Shahbazpour, and A. Olad, "pH sensitive and controlled release system based on cellulose nanofibers-poly vinyl alcohol hydrogels for cisplatin delivery," *Fibers Polym.*, vol. 18, no. 3, pp. 416–423, 2017.

[29] M. A. Casadei, G. Pitarresi, R. Calabrese, P. Paolicelli, and G. Giammona, "Biodegradable and pH-Sensitive hydrogels for potential colon-specific drug delivery : Characterization and in vitro release studies," *Biomacromolecules* pp. 43–49, 2008.

[30] S. Das and U. Subuddhi, "Cyclodextrin mediated controlled release of naproxen from pH-sensitive chitosan/poly(vinyl alcohol) hydrogels for colon targeted delivery," *Ind. Eng. Chem. Res.*, vol. 52, no. 39, pp. 14192–14200, 2013.

5555553322222111111111111111

[31] Y. Hu, Z. Mei, and X. Hu, "pH-sensitive interpenetrating network hydrogels based on pachyman and its carboxymethylated derivatives for oral drug delivery," *J. Polym. Res.*, vol. 22, no. 6, pp. 1–10, 2015.

[32] M. Fathi, M. Alami-Milani, M. H. Geranmayeh, J. Barar, H. Erfan-Niya, and Y. Omidi, "Dual thermo-and pH-sensitive injectable hydrogels of chitosan/(poly(N-isopropylacrylamide-co-itaconic acid)) for doxorubicin delivery in breast cancer," *Int. J. Biol. Macromol.*, vol. 128, pp. 957–964, 2019.

[33] V. R. Patel and M. M. Amiji, "pH-Sensitive swelling and drug-release properties of chitosan—poly(ethylene oxide) semi-interpenetrating polymer network," no. 9, *ACS Symposium Series* vol. 627, pp. 209–220, 2009.

[34] X. Qi *et al.*, "Salecan-based pH-sensitive hydrogels for insulin delivery," *Mol. Pharm.*, vol. 14, no. 2, pp. 431–440, 2017.

[35] S. Kunjiappan *et al.*, "Modeling a pH-sensitive Zein-co-acrylic acid hybrid hydrogels loaded 5-fluorouracil and rutin for enhanced anticancer efficacy by oral delivery," *3 Biotech*, vol. 9, no. 5, pp. 1–20, 2019.

[36] X. L. Wang, H. F. Yao, X. Y. Li, X. Wang, Y. P. Huang, and Z. S. Liu, "PH/temperature-sensitive hydrogel-based molecularly imprinted polymers (hydroMIPs) for drug delivery by frontal polymerization," *RSC Adv.*, vol. 6, no. 96, pp. 94038–94047, 2016.

[37] C. T. Huynh *et al.*, "Intraarterial gelation of injectable cationic pH/temperature-sensitive radiopaque embolic hydrogels in a rabbit hepatic tumor model and their potential application for liver cancer treatment," *RSC Adv.*, vol. 6, no. 53, pp. 47687–47697, 2016.

[38] C. Gao *et al.*, "Xylan-based temperature/pH sensitive hydrogels for drug controlled release," *Carbohydr. Polym.*, vol. 151, pp. 189–197, 2016.

[39] W. Zhang, X. Jin, H. Li, R. run Zhang, and C. wei Wu, "Injectable and body temperature sensitive hydrogels based on chitosan and hyaluronic acid for pH sensitive drug release," *Carbohydr. Polym.*, vol. 186, no. December 2017, pp. 82–90, 2018.

[40] D. Rafael *et al.*, "Sterilization procedure for temperature-sensitive hydrogels loaded with silver nanoparticles for clinical applications," *Nanomaterials*, vol. 9, no. 3, p. 380, 2019.

[41] S. Brahima, C. Boztepe, A. Kunkul, and M. Yuceer, "Modeling of drug release behavior of pH and temperature sensitive poly(NIPAAm-co-AAc) IPN hydrogels using response surface methodology and artificial neural networks," *Mater. Sci. Eng. C*, vol. 75, pp. 425–432, 2017.

[42] L. Zhang *et al.*, "Preparation of high-strength sustainable lignocellulose gels and their applications for antiultraviolet weathering and dye removal," *ACS Sustain. Chem. Eng.*, vol. 7, no. 3, pp. 2998–3009, 2019.

[43] S. Razani and A. Dadkhah Tehrani, "Development of new organic-inorganic, hybrid bionanocomposite from cellulose nanowhisker and Mg/Al-CO 3 -LDHfor enhanced dye removal," *Int. J. Biol. Macromol.*, vol. 133, pp. 892–901, 2019.

[44] Z. Yuan *et al.*, "Preparation of a poly(acrylic acid) based hydrogel with fast adsorption rate and high adsorption capacity for the removal of cationic dyes," *RSC Adv.*, vol. 9, no. 37, pp. 21075–21085, 2019.

[45] X. S. Hu, R. Liang, and G. Sun, "Super-adsorbent hydrogel for removal of methylene blue dye from aqueous solution," *J. Mater. Chem. A*, vol. 6, no. 36, pp. 17612–17624, 2018.

[46] M. Ranjbar-Mohammadi, M. Rahimdokht, and E. Pajootan, "Low cost hydrogels based on gum Tragacanth and TiO 2 nanoparticles: Characterization and RBFNN modelling of methylene blue dye removal," *Int. J. Biol. Macromol.*, vol. 134, pp. 967–975, 2019.

[47] X. Jv *et al.*, "Fabrication of a magnetic poly(aspartic acid)-poly(acrylic acid) hydrogel: Application for the adsorptive removal of organic dyes from aqueous solution," *J. Chem. Eng. Data*, vol. 64, no. 3, pp. 1228–1236, 2019.

[48] S. Huang, L. Wu, T. Li, D. Xu, X. Lin, and C. Wu, "Facile preparation of biomass lignin-based hydroxyethyl cellulose super-absorbent hydrogel for dye pollutant removal," *Int. J. Biol. Macromol.*, vol. 137, pp. 939–947, 2019.

[49] Ö. B. Üzüm, İ. Bayraktar, S. Kundakcı, and E. Karadağ, "Swelling behaviors of novel magnetic semi-IPN hydrogels and their application for Janus Green B removal," *Polym. Bull.*, no. 0123456789, 2019.

[50] N. Sezgin and N. Balkaya, "Removal of heavy metal ions from electroplating wastewater," *Desalin. Water Treat.*, vol. 93, pp. 257–266, 2017.

[51] T. Zeng *et al.*, "3D MnO 2 nanotubes@reduced graphene oxide hydrogel as reusable adsorbent for the removal of heavy metal ions," *Mater. Chem. Phys.*, vol. 231, no. April, pp. 105–108, 2019.

[52] S. Perumal, R. Atchudan, D. H. Yoon, J. Joo, and I. W. Cheong, "Spherical chitosan/gelatin hydrogel particles for removal of multiple heavy metal ions from wastewater," *Ind. Eng. Chem. Res.*, vol. 58, no. 23, pp. 9900–9907, 2019.

[53] G. He, C. Wang, J. Cao, L. Fan, S. Zhao, and Y. Chai, "Carboxymethyl chitosan-kaolinite composite hydrogel for efficient copper ions trapping," *J. Environ. Chem. Eng.*, vol. 7, no. 2, p. 102953, 2019.

[54] C. B. Godiya, M. Liang, S. M. Sayed, D. Li, and X. Lu, "Novel alginate/polyethyleneimine hydrogel adsorbent for cascaded removal and utilization of Cu 2+ and Pb 2+ ions," *J. Environ. Manage.*, vol. 232, no. August 2018, pp. 829–841, 2019.

[55] L. A. Shah *et al.*, "Superabsorbent polymer hydrogels with good thermal and mechanical properties for removal of selected heavy metal ions," *J. Clean. Prod.*, vol. 201, pp. 78–87, 2018.

[56] S. Lone, D. H. Yoon, H. Lee, and I. W. Cheong, "Gelatin-chitosan hydrogel particles for efficient removal of Hg(ii) from wastewater," *Environ. Sci. Water Res. Technol.*, vol. 5, no. 1, pp. 83–90, 2019.

[57] X. Wang *et al.*, "Permeable, robust and magnetic hydrogel beads: Water droplet templating synthesis and utilization for heavy metal ions removal," *J. Mater. Sci.*, vol. 53, no. 21, pp. 15009–15024, 2018.

[58] J. L. Guo, Y. S. Kim, and A. G. Mikos, "Biomacromolecules for tissue engineering: Emerging biomimetic strategies," *Biomacromolecules*, p. acs.biomac.9b00792, 2019.

[59] A. Mellati, S. Dai, J. Bi, B. Jin, and H. Zhang, "A biodegradable thermosensitive hydrogel with tuneable properties for mimicking three-dimensional microenvironments of stem cells," *RSC Adv.*, vol. 4, no. 109, pp. 63951–63961, 2014.

[60] B. Hermenegildo *et al.*, "Hydrogel-based magnetoelectric microenvironments for tissue stimulation," *Colloids Surfaces B Biointerfaces*, vol. 181, no. March, pp. 1041–1047, 2019.

[61] D. Xue, J. Zhang, Y. Wang, and D. Mei, "Digital light processing-based 3D printing of cell-seeding hydrogel scaffolds with regionally varied stiffness," *ACS Biomater. Sci. Eng.*, p. acsbiomaterials.9b00696, 2019.

[62] F. Ahadi, S. Khorshidi, and A. Karkhaneh, "A hydrogel/fiber scaffold based on silk fibroin/oxidized pectin with sustainable release of vancomycin hydrochloride," *Eur. Polym. J.*, vol. 118, no. June, pp. 265–274, 2019.

[63] X. Wu, S. I. Stroll, D. Lantigua, S. Suvarnapathaki, and G. Camci-Unal, "Eggshell particle-reinforced hydrogels for bone tissue engineering: An orthogonal approach," *Biomater. Sci.*, vol. 7, no. 7, pp. 2675–2685, 2019.

[64] E. Rederstorff *et al.*, "An in vitro study of two GAG-like marine polysaccharides incorporated into injectable hydrogels for bone and cartilage tissue engineering," *Acta Biomater.*, vol. 7, no. 5, pp. 2119–2130, 2011.

[65] D. N. Heo, M. Hospodiuk, and I. T. Ozbolat, "Synergistic interplay between human MSCs and HUVECs in 3D spheroids laden in collagen/fibrin hydrogels for bone tissue engineering," *Acta Biomater.*, no. xxxx, pp. 1–9, 2019.

[66] J. Fang, P. Li, X. Lu, L. Fang, X. Lü, and F. Ren, "A strong, tough, and osteoconductive hydroxyapatite mineralized polyacrylamide/dextran hydrogel for bone tissue regeneration," *Acta Biomater.*, vol. 88, pp. 503–513, 2019.

[67] A. Al-Sabah *et al.*, "Structural and mechanical characterization of crosslinked and sterilised nanocellulose-based hydrogels for cartilage tissue engineering," *Carbohydr. Polym.*, vol. 212, no. December 2018, pp. 242–251, 2019.

[68] S. H. Park *et al.*, "An injectable, click-crosslinked, cytomodulin-modified hyaluronic acid hydrogel for cartilage tissue engineering," *NPG Asia Mater.*, vol. 11, no. 1, pp. 1–16, 2019.

[69] F. You, B. F. Eames, and X. Chen, "Application of extrusion-based hydrogel bioprinting for cartilage tissue engineering," *Int. J. Mol. Sci.*, vol. 18, no. 7, pp. 8–14, 2017.

[70] G. C. J. Lindberg *et al.*, "Intact vitreous humor as a potential extracellular matrix hydrogel for cartilage tissue engineering applications," *Acta Biomater.*, vol. 85, pp. 117–130, 2019.

[71] B. A. Breen *et al.*, "Therapeutic effect of neurotrophin-3 treatment in an injectable collagen scaffold following rat spinal cord hemisection injury," *ACS Biomater. Sci. Eng.*, vol. 3, no. 7, pp. 1287–1295, 2017.

[72] L. M. Li *et al.*, "Peptide-tethered hydrogel scaffold promotes recovery from Spinal cord transection via synergism with mesenchymal stem cells," *ACS Appl. Mater. Interfaces*, vol. 9, no. 4, pp. 3330–3342, 2017.

[73] C. Chen *et al.*, "Bioinspired hydrogel electrospun fibers for spinal cord regeneration," *Adv. Funct. Mater.*, vol. 29, no. 4, pp. 1–11, 2019.

[74] K. Qiao *et al.*, "Effects of graphene on the structure, properties, electro-response behaviors of GO/PAA composite hydrogels and influence of electro-mechanical coupling on BMSC differentiation," *Mater. Sci. Eng. C*, vol. 93, no. August, pp. 853–863, 2018.

[75] N. Mauro *et al.*, "Degradable poly(amidoamine) hydrogels as scaffolds for in vitro culturing of peripheral nervous system cells," *Macromol. Biosci.*, vol. 13, no. 3, pp. 332–347, 2013.

[76] P. Sekar and A. Chauhan, "Effect of vitamin-E integration on delivery of prostaglandin analogs from therapeutic lenses," *J. Colloid Interface Sci.*, vol. 539, pp. 457–467, 2019.

[77] I. Postic and H. Sheardown, "Altering the release of tobramycin by incorporating poly(ethylene glycol) into model silicone hydrogel contact lens materials," *J. Biomater. Sci. Polym. Ed.*, vol. 30, no. 13, pp. 1115–1141, 2019.

[78] S. Wei *et al.*, "Gas-permeable, irritation-free, transparent hydrogel contact lens devices with metal-coated nanofiber mesh for eye interfacing," *ACS Nano*, vol. 13, pp. 7920–7929, 2019.

[79] W. Yan-long., "Synthesis and characterization of silicone hydrogel contact lens materials." *Applied Chemical Industry*, 2, pp.316–318, 2014.

[80] Y. Wu, D. Wang, I. Willner, Y. Tian, and L. Jiang, "Smart DNA hydrogel integrated nanochannels with high ion flux and adjustable selective ionic transport," *Angew. Chemie—Int. Ed.*, vol. 57, no. 26, pp. 7790–7794, 2018.

[81] N. Ren *et al.*, "DNA-based hybrid hydrogels sustain water-insoluble ophthalmic therapeutic delivery against allergic conjunctivitis," *ACS Appl. Mater. Interfaces*, vol. 11, no. 30, pp. 26704–26710, 2019.

[82] J. Nam, W. S. Jang, J. Kim, H. Lee, and C. S. Lim, "Lamb wave-based molecular diagnosis using DNA hydrogel formation by rolling circle amplification (RCA) process," *Biosens. Bioelectron.*, vol. 142, no. July, p. 111496, 2019.

[83] Y. Lin *et al.*, "A chemiluminescent biosensor for ultrasensitive detection of adenosine based on target-responsive DNA hydrogel with Au@HKUST-1 encapsulation," *Sensors Actuators, B Chem.*, vol. 289, no. March, pp. 56–64, 2019.

[84] K. Abe, I. Kawamata, S. I. M. Nomura, and S. Murata, "Programmable reactions and diffusion using DNA for pattern formation in hydrogel medium," *Mol. Syst. Des. Eng.*, vol. 4, no. 3, pp. 639–643, 2019.

[85] C. Li, H. Li, J. Ge, and G. Jie, "Versatile fluorescence detection of microRNA based on novel DNA hydrogel-amplified signal probes coupled with DNA walker amplification," *Chem. Commun.*, vol. 55, no. 27, pp. 3919–3922, 2019.

3 Conducting Polymer-Based Hydrogels and Scaffolds

Neha Kanwar Rawat and Anujit Ghosal

CONTENTS

3.1 INTRODUCTION

Conducting polymers (CPs) were first reported in the mid-1970s as a new generation of organic materials that have both electrical and optical properties like those of metals and inorganic semiconductors [1, 2]. They also have attractive features that make them significant like the ease of synthesis and flexibility in processing over conventional polymers [3, 4]. CPs find vast applications including fuel cells, computer displays, supercapacitors, corrosion-resistant coatings, and many others [5–8]. CPs can be synthesized alone as polymers or as interpenetrating polymer networks, composites, hybrids, and nanostructured materials with conferred biodegradability and biocompatibility [9]. They are electroactive as well as conducting in nature, exhibiting properties requisite for biomaterials which can be used for electro-response applications. They can bind to biologically significant molecules prior to functionalization, and, thus, their properties can be improved for further advanced applications. CPs exhibit a combination of properties possessed by metals and conventional polymers—i.e., showing the potential to conduct charge, excellent electrical as well as optical properties, accompanying flexibility, and ease in synthesis and processing. CPs can also attain high conductivity by the phenomenon of "doping". The family "polyheterocycles" contains the

CPs of interest to researchers, e.g., polypyrrole, polyaniline, polythiophene, and their derivatives. A brief classification of CPs based on their synthesis, properties, and applications has been drafted in Figure 3.1. As they are conducting in nature, they can be utilized in drug release, biosensors, tissue engineering, stimuli-responsive biomimetic polymeric materials, and other such medical applications [10]. In light of the fact that several tissues are responsive to electrical fields and stimuli, CPs have attracted great potential for several biological and medical applications [11].

The conducting polymers conduct electricity due to their ability to adjust/modify into various electronic forms. Examples of polyaniline (PANI) CP in different forms are presented in Figure 3.2. The synthetic macromolecule possessing a highly delocalized π-conjugated backbone structure and configurable side chains allows the CPs to conduct, otherwise it may not (Figure 3.2A in comparison to B–D).

The variation in ionic forms or number π-conjugated delocalized electron alters the conductivity of the CPs [12, 13]. Some of the most common examples of CPs are polyacetylene (PA), polypyrrole (PPy), polyaniline (PANI), polythiophene (PTh), poly (3,4-ethylenedioxythiophene) (PEDOT), polyfluorenes (PF), poly(p-phenylene vinylene) (PPV), poly(phenylene) (PPP), poly(p-phenylene ethynylene) (PPE), and their derivatives. Structurally, the CP backbone is made of alternating single C-C, double C=C, or triple C≡C bonds. The highly delocalized electrons are weakly held together by π bonds whereas the overall polymeric chain strength is regulated by the strong σ bonds. The conjugated double or triple bonds along their backbone are primarily responsible for the exceptional electrical conductivity displayed by CPs. Furthermore, this conjugated backbone architecture endows CPs with other unique electronic and photo-physical properties, such as tunable electron affinity and ionization energy as well as high conductivity. The significant features by which CPs have been useful for the biomedical field include,

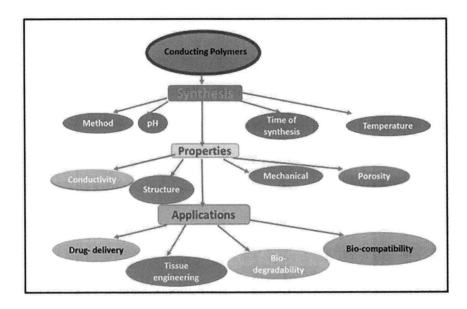

FIGURE 3.1   Classification of CPs on the basis of their synthesis, properties, and applications.

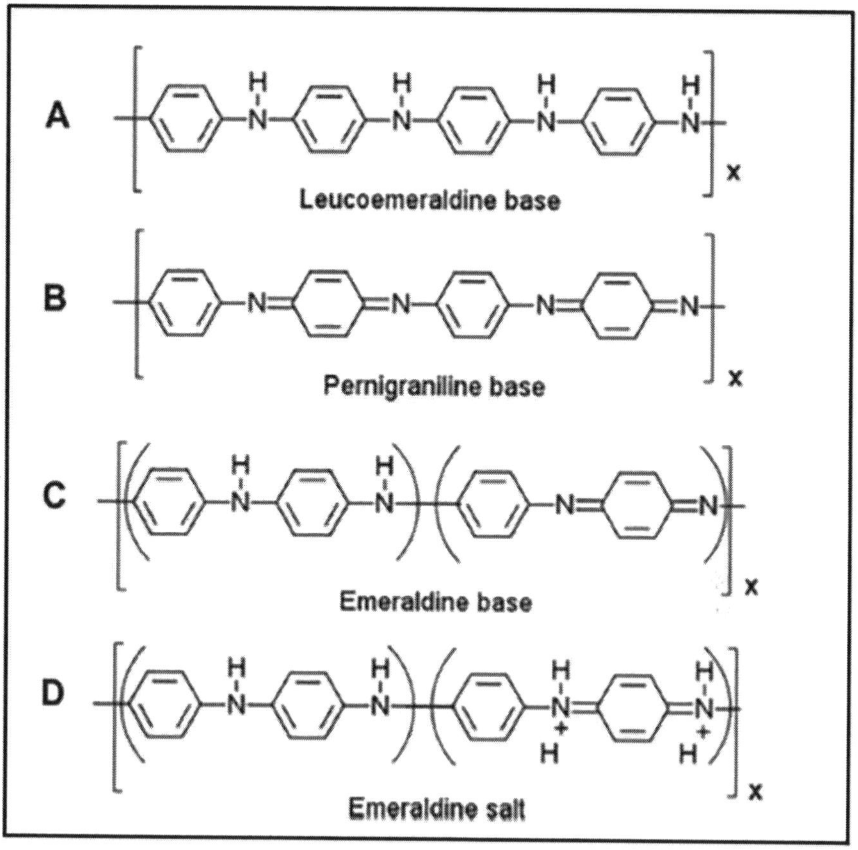

FIGURE 3.2 Showing various electronic states of PANI.

prominently, biocompatibility; their control and release behavior (i.e., reversible doping); their charge transfer capability, and, above all, their varying compatibility [14].

3.2 CLASSIFICATION OF CONDUCTING POLYMERS AND THEIR SPECIFIC BIOMEDICAL APPLICATIONS

Among the growing importance of CPs, PANI has mainly fueled the speedy development of this unique class of polymers in recent years. Table 3.1 lists a few of the CPs and their application fields with prominent research references [15–22].

3.2.1 POLYANILINE

The most explored CPs are polyaniline (PANI) or aniline black and are also the easiest to synthesize. It occurs in three states: one as pernigraniline base, which is fully oxidized; the emeraldine base, which is half oxidized intermediate state (conducting

TABLE 3.1

Biomedical Applications of Some CPs With Their Properties Supporting Their Biomedical Use

Composite/blend	Conductivity (S/cm)	Properties	Suggested applications	Prominent reviews	Ref.
PEDOT:PSS/PU (aqueous dispersion)	More than 110–120	Electrically promising	Tactile skin-based sensors	Ding et al.	[15]
Polythiophene derivative/PU		Promising photophysical property	Suitable for supporting electrically stimulated cell growth	Jea et al.	[16]
PANI nanofibre/ bacterial cellulose	10^{-2}	Good cell-line studies	Bone regeneration, tissue engineering	Wang et al.	[17]
PAni nanoparticles/ poly(acrylic acid)/ polyvinyl alcohol	10^{-2}	Flexible, Sterchable	Tissue engineering	Broda et al.	[18]
PPy nanoparticles/PU		Stretchable, stress-strain sensors	Human health by motion detection	Mufang et al.	[19]
PPy/poly(D,L-lactic acid)	10^{-3}		NMR magnetic resonance imaging	Jaymand et al.	[20]
Polythiophene-Polycaprolactone	Decreased conductivity as compared to neat PTh	Scaffolds	Tissue engineering	Maryam et al.	[21]
Collagen/alginate/ polypyrrole hydrogels	118.37	Hydrogels	Cell-line studies	Farinaz et al.	[22]

out of three); and the third, leucoemeraldine base, is sufficiently reduced (Figure 3.2) [23]. The different forms of PANI, mainly the conducting kind (PANI hydrochloride), have more favorable properties than the non-conducting type (emeraldine base). PANI has a very vast application in the biomedical field, as reports depict, owing to its facile synthesis and high conducting nature. Although a few shortcomings, such as the difficulty in easy processability and, above all, poor properties like flexibility, degradability, and cell compatibility, restrict its vast application in the field. Literature reports depict chronic inflammation once implanted in several animal studies. Particularly, the virgin applications of PANI are greatly hampered in the biomedical arena. However, the versatile tailored properties of PANI have been studied via in vivo animal modeling methods to verify the applicability of PANI in this field for future escalation to human applications. All such drawbacks of respective CPs can be overcome or balanced by composite formation with inorganic or organic components [8, 14, 24, 25]. In other prominent methods to develop biomedical usage of PANI, it was studied in combination with biodegradable polymers which serve as hosts to form biocomposites possessing advanced mechanical, electrical, and surface properties [26]. Recent reports show conducting PANI and its derivatives can elicit favorable response from different cell lines under electrical stimuli and form novel biomaterials for bioengineering, particularly for tissues and organs showing electrical signals [27]. Some research groups have been working on making composites of PANI grafted with biodegradable electroactive polymers like gelatin and genipin [28]. The cross-linking leads to the formation of biodegradable electroactive hydrogels in cell therapy for native cardiac tissues with moderate electrical conductivity [29]. Such hydrogels have shown positive degradability studies when tested for 7 to 14 days with significant weight loss of about 50% to 60% in pH 7.4 at 37°C [20]. Biocompatible hydrogel-based sensors have been prepared using PANI and poly(acrylamide-co-hydroxyethyl methyl acrylate) (P(AAm-co-HEMA)) interpenetrating networks (Figure 3.3).

The same has been used as a strain and vibration sensor to be used as an electronic skin or wearable sensor/platform (Figure 3.4). Such promising results have motivated the research of CPs in hydrogels for direct or indirect biomedical applications [30].

3.2.2 POLYPYRROLE

Polypyrrole (PPy) has shown the best results when tissue engineering as far as clinical applications are concerned [22]. This conducting polymer shows promising properties when studied under physiological conditions. The main functions include biocompatibility (both in vitro and in vivo) and their ease of converting charges across the polymer backbone, which is needed in chemical reactions for biological processes. The doping characteristic to release and entrap biological molecules that match the generated electrical signals to varying outputs designed for medical The characteristic of the doped material is designed to release and entrap biological molecules/ drug (on demand) triggered by varying electrical signal outputs for medical applications like neural probes, nerve drug delivery devices, magnetic imaging, etc. [31–33]. All these advantages can be easily achieved by covalent insertion of various functional groups into the main PPy backbone, along with some necessary

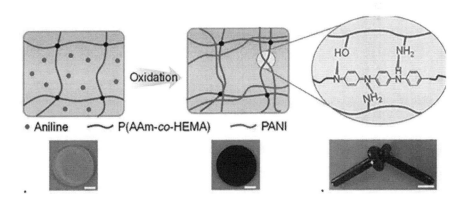

FIGURE 3.3 Schematic illustration of the synthesis of interpenetrating PANI/P(AAm-co-HEMA) hydrogels. Scale bars: 2 cm [30].

Source: Copyright permission from ACS (American Chemical Society).

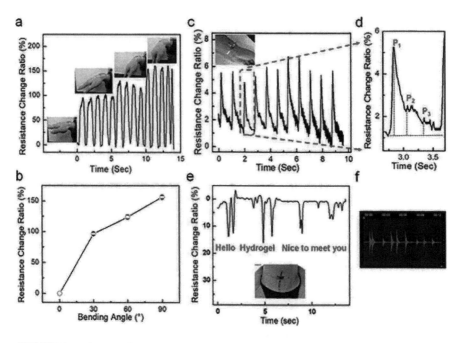

FIGURE 3.4 Signals from hydrogel sensors (a) on the wrist cyclically bending (b) as a function of bending angle, (c, d) on the wrist pulse, and (e) on the throat of a volunteer speaking "Hello", "Hydrogel" and "Nice to meet you", in comparison to (f) the same voice wave recorded using a smartphone [30].

Source: Copyright permission from ACS.

adjustments in physical and chemical properties including redox (charge) stability, doping-de-doping, roughness, porosity, hydrophobicity, degradation, and conductivity. PPy also shows excellent chemical stability (in air and water) under physiological conditions [34]. PPy has one heteroatom position which it can use for extending its chain by combining with other functional groups, and these enhance the interaction/interface with biological molecules. The main advantage of using PPy is the easy preparation of the large surface areas, which has varying porosities and can be altered easily. These advantages make it beneficial for biomedical applications by giving advantageous permeability to bioactive molecules on its surface. PPy cannot be used in its pure forms as it is deficient in strength in nature and not useful for biomedical applications. Thus, copolymers with other polymers as wells composites can be used instead. PPy has numerous applications in biosensors, tissue engineering, drug delivery systems, implants, scaffolds, neural probes, and others [18, 33, 35].

3.2.3 Polythiophene

Polythiophene (PTh) is one of the polymers having sulphur as a heteroatom included in its cyclic chain with a higher conductivity as its prominent asset. The derivatives of PTh are highly explored for biomedical and other applications. One of the interesting members of the PTh family is poly(3,4-ethylenedioxythiophene) (PEDOT), which is formed by the polymerization of bicyclic monomer 3,4-ethylenedioxythiophene [36–38]. Research on this material depicts that it has become the most significant CP, possessing extraordinary properties like electrical, thermal, chemical, and high conductivity. It is used prominently in varying biomedical areas like nervous system devices, heart patches, and other drug delivery systems. Yasin et al., for the first time, fabricated porous PEDOT structures via the sacrificial colloidal template [39]. These nanostructures have advanced properties like enhanced surface area, decreased impedance values, and minimum cytotoxicity behavior. These also help in maintaining good redox cycles, which helps in making biomedical devices, biosensing, and drug delivery. Sequiera et al. fabricated nanostructured PEDOT and its composite with starch/κ-carrageenan aerogels as templates. κ-carrageenan is a biopolymer that acts as a doping agent for PEDOT CP and helps in increasing conductivity and finally enhances the electrical signals response. This doped PEDOT with κ-carrageenan leads to highly conducting PEDOT nanostructures with favorable properties for biomedical applications [40]. Another prominent derivative of PTh is poly(3-hexylthiophene), which has good biomedical and photovoltaic applications [41–44]. The positive advantageous side group present makes it an important member, leading to better solubility in organic solvents and electrical conductivity. Therefore, it shows better suitability to the nature of the specific biomedical applications. These include biosensors, neural probes, drug delivery devices, tissue engineering scaffolds, and bioactuators. Figure 3.5 shows the fabrication of nanoweb

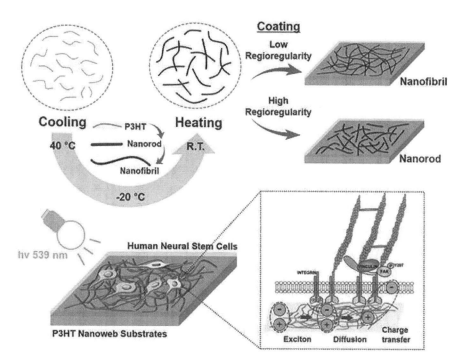

FIGURE 3.5 Schematic illustration of fabrication and application of photoelectric poly(3-hexylthiophene) (P3HT) nanoweb substrates for enhancing neuronal differentiation of human fetal neural stem cells (hfNSCs) [45].

substrate for differentiation of neural stem cells which at the latter stage can be developed for neuroengineering [45]. The conductive substrate was chosen for optoelectrical stimulation of stem cells neurogenesis. The effect of variation in temperature on the self-assembly process of the CPs, pulsed optoelectrical stimulation, and the focal adhesion development variation on assemblies, i.e. nanofibrils and nanorods for differentiation of human fetal neural stem cells, was explained [45].

PTh-based CPs and their derivatives show numerous usages in biomedical applications mainly in biocompatibility and the entrapping capability of varying biomolecules on their surface, as well as all reversing doping-de-doping phenomenon. They also have inbuilt capability due to their high conductivity and show positive biological responses from various cell lines, which respond to electrical stimuli from varying human body organs; therefore, they are well designed for biological tissues and internal body organs [41].

3.3 APPLICATIONS OF CPS IN THE BIOMEDICAL ARENA

CPs have become a distinctive family of polymeric materials with chemical, electrical, and biological properties. The promising advanced properties make this area more challenging and therefore, may lead to the design and development of advanced materials for various biomedical areas like tissue engineering regenerative medicine, biomedical imaging, biomedical implants, bioelectronics devices, and consumer electronics. In this section, we will discuss the application aspects of CPs in the varying biomedical fields discussed prior.

3.3.1 HYDROGELS

CPs having tremendous outstanding properties have some basic disadvantages in flexibility and mechanical strength. Thus, these anomalies can be improved by the formation of CP-based hydrogel blends. Hydrogels are unique materials that can absorb and retain large quantities of water, even more than the human body. The formation of blends based on CP hydrogels gives all the improvement in mechanical properties like stretchability and bendability along with a basic platform for bioactive agents. CP has been found to perform more efficiently as composites or blends in which hydrogels have the best properties. The significant properties include their lightweight, elastic, and conductive spongy behavior, with excellent stress-sensing characteristics. Hence, they are best termed as excellent tissue engineering precursor materials [11, 46–48].

The main method of formation of CP-based hydrogels is either by polymerization forming networks inside gels or by dispersion or via another known process of dehydration. In the latter water is removed from the gel and then CP is encapsulated inside, followed by a re-swelling of monomer in CPs. The main function of using CP in hydrogels-based systems is the formation of one continuous phase. However, the electrical conductivity values decrease when these hydrogels start leaching out of the host matrix to make electron-transferring domains.

The CP-based biosensors have emerged as the most significant because they have the requisite condition of mandatory minimum conductivity values to fabricate electrode materials. These electrodes are the main components of hydrogels-based biosensors. They also have high charge-discharge capability viz. redox cycles and basic flexibility that hydrogels need [49]. These conducting hydrogels can be created with favorable properties as discussed prior, which allows binding to bioactive molecules at specific locations inside the human body [49, 50]. They also find applications in drug release devices and brain stimulators. Electroconductive hydrogels have been used for the detection of vitamins, glucose, human metabolites, cell viability and function, lactate, DNA, dopamine, peptide, tumors, and hydrogen peroxide. Hydrogels produced electrochemically by growing PPy within poly(2-hydroxyethyl methacrylate) and poly(2-methoxy-5-aniline sulfonic acid) as dopant are reported to have high surface area and lower impedance relative to PPy film. Other examples involve PPy and mucopolysaccharide hydrogels, which are non-toxic and can be employed for drug release and neural and tissue engineering [9, 51, 52].

3.3.2 TISSUE ENGINEERING AND REGENERATIVE MEDICINE

The application of CPs started at an early stage in arenas of tissue engineering and regenerative medicine. Their application here owes to their promising properties like high electrical conductivity, controlled biodegradability, redox stability, and three-dimensional structural flexibility. The main tissue engineering application for a decade is seen in curing physiological disorders with long-lasting and devastating impacts. These are mainly related to various nervous, spinal, and bone defects, injuries, and deformations. The requisite condition of tissue engineering leads to the formation of complex native cellular environments using various multiple tasks aptly known as biomaterials. The mechanism of these scaffolds fabricated from CPs having properties similar to host tissues comes from their certain extraordinary properties, such as the ability to stimulate most cellular and tissue behaviors, proliferation, differentiation, cellular adhesion, and tissue formation. The other important factor to be considered is biodegradability, as old tissue scaffolds have to be replaced with new ones with passage of time, to make them skilled in expediting these novel cell-biomaterial interfaces. Literature depicts that both natural and synthetic polymer are used in fabrication of biomaterials for tissue engineering scaffolds and regenerative medicines [46, 50, 53].

3.3.3 DRUG DELIVERY

One of the most unique applications of CPs in the biological arena is drug delivery. Drug delivery signifies formulations and technologies for transporting macromolecules with biological significance. The bioactive molecule needs to be released at a particular microenvironment at a particular dose rate. CPs are redox-active materials with tunable electronic and physical properties. The charge of the CP backbone can be manipulated through redox processes with the accompanied movement of ions into and out of the polymer to maintain electrostatic neutrality. CPs with defined micro- or nanostructures have greatly enhanced surface areas compared to conventionally prepared CPs. The resulting high surface area interfaces between polymer and liquid media facilities ion exchange and can lead to larger and more rapid responses to redox cycling. CP systems are maturing as platforms for electrically tunable drug delivery. CPs with defined micro- or nanostructures offer the ability to increase the amount of drug that can be delivered while enabling systems to be finely tuned to control the extent and rate of drug release. This method of drug delivery has been increasing, yet it has some challenges to face, one being the controlled delivery to a patient or specific body parts. This anomaly has been successfully solved by the use of CPs and their many promising properties, such as high porosity, high charge density across polymeric chains, and binding ability to bound molecules over them. The control and release behavior of these biomolecules through redox behavior over CPs leads to drug release. Thus, varying therapeutic drugs which help stimulate proper nervous system growth, such as heparin, dopamine, and naproxen, had been positively implanted with help of CPs. PEDOT has been used for the delivery of ibuprofen (ionic form). There are certain drawbacks such as leaching of bound molecules, the fatigue of CPs, swelling/deswelling, pits/decrements, delamination, and degradation of the polymer [25, 54–56].

3.4 BIOMEDICAL COMPOSITES

The overall improvement and complete application of CPs for biomedical applications are only possible if we totally eradicate the toxicity or adverse effect of CPs. The most suitable way of achieving this is the development of composite materials using CPs and other suitable additives [56–60]. A composite is a final product of a combination of two or more different materials. The outcome is considered and mostly more advanced (often stronger) than the individual components. The biomedical application needs very close estimation of the constituent parts due to probable individual health hazardous effects. The most prominent method to enhance the application of CPs in the biomedical field is to make their composites with other materials. This methodology certainly removes the probable shortcomings of CPs, and the synergistic properties of the biopolymer generally mask any harmful effects of CPs. The composite formation also overcomes the dispersibility of the CPs in an aqueous system. Mawad et al. developed a novel CP-based electroactive system with very high conductivity of 2.7×10^{-2} S cm^{-1} with erodible nature [5, 61]. Promisingly, these materials were found to stimulate cell adhesion, growth, cytocompatibility, and possible tailored properties. PPy when combined with poly(D, L-lactide)-based composites also leads to improved conductivity. The conducting system behaves positively on animal models showing only minor inflammation (with rats), with the PANI being the most common CP, yet it is less explored compared to other CPs. However, few prominent reports of PANI and its copolymers, i.e., poly(aniline-co-ethyl-3-aminobenzoate) and poly (aniline-co-3aminobenzoic acid), used in biomedical applications have been reported [62–64].

3.5 CONCLUSIONS

CP-based hydrogels have marvelous applications in the biomedical arena, including tissue engineering, but more work is still required for a high level of certainty. The novel synthesized CPs, having multi-functional properties, can be widely used for human health benefits. The increased ability of binding large amounts of molecules and releasing them in a controllable mode makes these materials potential drug delivery agents facilitating neurotissue engineering processes. All modifications rely on the utmost parameter that defines the uniqueness of CPs: their conductivity and compatibility with the host matrix. This ever-growing field needs a lot of innovations and continuous progress for delivering the product with utmost importance in the field of biomedicine.

REFERENCES

[1] P. Chandrasekhar, Conducting polymers, *Fundamentals and Applications*, (1999).

[2] H. Yoon, J. Jang, Conducting-polymer nanomaterials for high-performance sensor applications: Issues and challenges, *Advanced Functional Materials*, 19 (2009) 1567–1576.

[3] P.J. Nigrey, A.G. MacDiarmid, A.J. Heeger, Electrochemistry of polyacetylene,(CH) x: electrochemical doping of (CH) x films to the metallic state, *Journal of the Chemical Society, Chemical Communications* (1979) 594–595.

[4] H. Shirakawa, E.J. Louis, A.G. MacDiarmid, C.K. Chiang, A.J. Heeger, Synthesis of electrically conducting organic polymers: halogen derivatives of polyacetylene,(CH) x, *Journal of the Chemical Society, Chemical Communications* (1977) 578–580.

[5] D. Mawad, A. Lauto, G.G. Wallace, Conductive polymer hydrogels, in: *Polymeric Hydrogels as Smart Biomaterials*, Springer, Switzerland 2016, pp. 19–44.

[6] T-H. Le, Y. Kim, H. Yoon, Electrical and electrochemical properties of conducting polymers, *Polymers*, 9 (2017) 150.

[7] H. Khatoon, S. Iqbal, S. Ahmad, Conductive thermoset composites, thermoset composites: Preparation, *Properties and Applications*, 38 (2018) 189.

[8] N.K. Rawat, A. Ghosal, S. Ahmad, Influence of microwave irradiation on various properties of nanopolythiophene and their anticorrosive nanocomposite coatings, *RSC Advances*, 4 (2014) 50594–50605.

[9] R. Balint, N.J. Cassidy, S.H. Cartmell, Conductive polymers: Towards a smart biomaterial for tissue engineering, *Acta Biomaterialia*, 10 (2014) 2341–2353.

[10] Kenry, B. Liu, Recent advances in biodegradable conducting polymers and their biomedical applications, *Biomacromolecules*, 19 (2018) 1783–1803.

[11] B. Guo, P.X. Ma, Conducting polymers for tissue engineering, *Biomacromolecules*, 19 (2018) 1764–1782.

[12] S.I. Cho, S.B. Lee, Fast electrochemistry of conductive polymer nanotubes: Synthesis, mechanism, and application, *Accounts of Chemical Research*, 41 (2008) 699–707.

[13] A. Monkman, D. Bloor, G. Stevens, J. Stevens, P. Wilson, Electronic structure and charge transport mechanisms in polyaniline, *Synthetic Metals*, 29 (1989) 277–284.

[14] N.K. Rawat, S. Ahmad, P. Panda, Influence of boron incorporation on poly (phenyldiammine) nanostructures: Novel, well-defined and highly conducting nanospheres dispersed smart corrosion protective epoxy coatings, *Composites Communications*, 9 (2018) 81–85.

[15] P. Tang, G. Hu, Y. Gao, W. Li, S. Yao, Z. Liu, D. Ma, The microwave adsorption behavior and microwave-assisted heteroatoms doping of graphene-based nano-carbon materials, *Scientific Reports*, 4 (2014) 5901.

[16] J.W. Jo, J.W. Jung, H-W. Wang, P. Kim, T.P. Russell, W.H. Jo, Fluorination of polythiophene derivatives for high performance organic photovoltaics, *Chemistry of Materials*, 26 (2014) 4214–4220.

[17] H. Wang, E. Zhu, J. Yang, P. Zhou, D. Sun, W. Tang, Bacterial cellulose nanofiber-supported polyaniline nanocomposites with flake-shaped morphology as supercapacitor electrodes, *The Journal of Physical Chemistry C*, 116 (2012) 13013–13019.

[18] C.R. Broda, J.Y. Lee, S. Sirivisoot, C.E. Schmidt, B.S. Harrison, A chemically polymerized electrically conducting composite of polypyrrole nanoparticles and polyurethane for tissue engineering, *Journal of Biomedical Materials Research Part A*, 98 (2011) 509–516.

[19] M. Li, H. Li, W. Zhong, Q. Zhao, D. Wang, Stretchable conductive polypyrrole/polyurethane (PPy/PU) strain sensor with netlike microcracks for human breath detection, *ACS Applied Materials & Interfaces*, 6 (2014) 1313–1319.

[20] M. Jaymand, R. Sarvari, P. Abbaszadeh, B. Massoumi, M. Eskandani, Y. Beygi-Khosrowshahi, Development of novel electrically conductive scaffold based on hyperbranched polyester and polythiophene for tissue engineering applications, *Journal of Biomedical Materials Research Part A*, 104 (2016) 2673–2684.

[21] M. Hatamzadeh, P. Najafi-Moghadam, A. Baradar-Khoshfetrat, M. Jaymand, B. Massoumi, Novel nanofibrous electrically conductive scaffolds based on poly (ethylene glycol) s-modified polythiophene and poly (ε-caprolactone) for tissue engineering applications, *Polymer*, 107 (2016) 177–190.

[22] F. Ketabat, A. Karkhaneh, R. Mehdinavaz Aghdam, S. Hossein Ahmadi Tafti, Injectable conductive collagen/alginate/polypyrrole hydrogels as a biocompatible system for biomedical applications, *Journal of Biomaterials Science, Polymer Edition*, 28 (2017) 794–805.

[23] S. Bhadra, D. Khastgir, N.K. Singha, J.H. Lee, Progress in preparation, processing and applications of polyaniline, *Progress in Polymer Science*, 34 (2009) 783–810.

[24] Y. Zhang, L. Lin, Z. Feng, J. Zhou, Z. Lin, Fabrication of a PANI/Au nanocomposite modified nanoelectrode for sensitive dopamine nanosensor design, *Electrochimica Acta*, 55 (2009) 265–270.

[25] A. Ghosal, S. Tiwari, A. Mishra, A. Vashist, N.K. Rawat, S. Ahmad, J. Bhattacharya, Design and engineering of nanogels, in: *Nanogels for Biomedical Applications*, book by (Royal society of chemistry) RSC publications 2017, pp. 9–28.

[26] S. Meer, A. Kausar, T. Iqbal, Trends in conducting polymer and hybrids of conducting polymer/carbon nanotube: A review, *Polymer-Plastics Technology and Engineering*, 55 (2016) 1416–1440.

[27] T.H. Qazi, R. Rai, A.R. Boccaccini, Tissue engineering of electrically responsive tissues using polyaniline based polymers: A review, *Biomaterials*, 35 (2014) 9068–9086.

[28] L. Li, J. Ge, P.X. Ma, B. Guo, Injectable conducting interpenetrating polymer network hydrogels from gelatin-graft-polyaniline and oxidized dextran with enhanced mechanical properties, *RSC Advances*, 5 (2015) 92490–92498.

[29] R. Dong, X. Zhao, B. Guo, P.X. Ma, Self-healing conductive injectable hydrogels with antibacterial activity as cell delivery carrier for cardiac cell therapy, *ACS Applied Materials & Interfaces*, 8 (2016) 17138–17150.

[30] Z. Wang, J. Chen, Y. Cong, H. Zhang, T. Xu, L. Nie, J. Fu, Ultrastretchable strain sensors and arrays with high sensitivity and linearity based on super tough conductive hydrogels, *Chemistry of Materials*, 30 (2018) 8062–8069.

[31] D.H. Kim, S.M. Richardson-Burns, J.L. Hendricks, C. Sequera, D.C. Martin, Effect of immobilized nerve growth factor on conductive polymers: Electrical properties and cellular response, *Advanced Functional Materials*, 17 (2007) 79–86.

[32] X. Cui, J.F. Hetke, J.A. Wiler, D.J. Anderson, D.C. Martin, Electrochemical deposition and characterization of conducting polymer polypyrrole/PSS on multichannel neural probes, *Sensors and Actuators A: Physical*, 93 (2001) 8–18.

[33] X. Song, H. Gong, S. Yin, L. Cheng, C. Wang, Z. Li, Y. Li, X. Wang, G. Liu, Z. Liu, Ultra-small iron oxide doped polypyrrole nanoparticles for in vivo multimodal imaging guided photothermal therapy, *Advanced Functional Materials*, 24 (2014) 1194–1201.

[34] Y. Wei, B. Li, C. Fu, H. Qi, Electroactive conducting polymers for biomedical applications, *Acta Polymerica Sinica*, 12 (2010) 1399–1405.

[35] J.Y. Lee, C.A. Bashur, A.S. Goldstein, C.E. Schmidt, Polypyrrole-coated electrospun PLGA nanofibers for neural tissue applications, *Biomaterials*, 30 (2009) 4325–4335.

[36] P. Kinlen, D. Silverman, C. Jeffreys, Corrosion protection using polyanujne coating formulations, *Synthetic Metals*, 85 (1997) 1327–1332.

[37] E.W.C. Chan, D. Bennet, P. Baek, D. Barker, S. Kim, J. Travas-Sejdic, Electrospun polythiophene phenylenes for tissue engineering, *Biomacromolecules*, 19 (2018) 1456–1468.

[38] C. Xu, S. Guan, S. Wang, W. Gong, T. Liu, X. Ma, C. Sun, Biodegradable and electroconductive poly (3, 4-ethylenedioxythiophene)/carboxymethyl chitosan hydrogels for neural tissue engineering, *Materials Science and Engineering: C*, 84 (2018) 32–43.

[39] M.N. Yasin, R.K. Brooke, S. Rudd, A. Chan, W-T. Chen, G.I. Waterhouse, D. Evans, I.D. Rupenthal, D. Svirskis, 3-Dimensionally ordered macroporous PEDOT ion-exchange resins prepared by vapor phase polymerization for triggered drug delivery: Fabrication and characterization, *Electrochimica Acta*, 269 (2018) 560–570.

[40] R. Zamora-Sequeira, I. Ardao, R. Starbird, C.A. García-González, Conductive nanostructured materials based on poly-(3, 4-ethylenedioxythiophene)(PEDOT) and starch/κ-carrageenan for biomedical applications, *Carbohydrate Polymers*, 189 (2018) 304–312.

[41] C. Garcia-Escobar, M. Nicho, H. Hu, G. Alvarado-Tenorio, P. Altuzar-Coello, G. Cadenas-Pliego, D. Hernandez-Martinez, Effect of microwave radiation on the synthesis of poly (3-hexylthiophene) and the subsequent photovoltaic performance of CdS/P3HT solar cells, *International Journal of Polymer Science* vol 2016, Article ID 1926972, pp-1-9 (2016).

[42] S.W. Lee, H.J. Lee, J.H. Choi, W.G. Koh, J.M. Myoung, J.H. Hur, J.J. Park, J.H. Cho, U. Jeong, Periodic array of polyelectrolyte-gated organic transistors from electrospun poly (3-hexylthiophene) nanofibers, *Nano Letters*, 10 (2009) 347–351.

[43] B.K. Kuila, A. Garai, A.K. Nandi, Synthesis, optical, and electrical characterization of organically soluble silver nanoparticles and their poly (3-hexylthiophene) nanocomposites: Enhanced luminescence property in the nanocomposite thin films, *Chemistry of Materials*, 19 (2007) 5443–5452.

[44] K. Yang, J.Y. Oh, J.S. Lee, Y. Jin, G-E. Chang, S.S. Chae, E. Cheong, H.K. Baik, S-W. Cho, Photoactive poly (3-hexylthiophene) nanoweb for optoelectrical stimulation to enhance neurogenesis of human stem cells, *Theranostics*, 7 (2017) 4591.

[45] K. Yang, J.Y. Oh, J.S. Lee, Y. Jin, G-E. Chang, S.S. Chae, E. Cheong, H.K. Baik, S-W. Cho, Photoactive poly(3-hexylthiophene) nanoweb for optoelectrical stimulation to enhance neurogenesis of human stem cells, *Theranostics*, 7 (2017) 4591–4604.

[46] M. Talikowska, X. Fu, G. Lisak, Application of conducting polymers to wound care and skin tissue engineering: A review, *Biosensors and Bioelectronics*, 135 (2019) 50–63.

[47] I. Noshadi, B.W. Walker, R. Portillo-Lara, E. Shirzaei Sani, N. Gomes, M.R. Aziziyan, N. Annabi, Engineering biodegradable and biocompatible bio-ionic liquid conjugated hydrogels with tunable conductivity and mechanical properties, *Scientific Reports*, 7 (2017) 4345.

[48] M. Uz, S.K. Mallapragada, Conductive polymers and hydrogels for neural tissue engineering, *Journal of the Indian Institute of Science*, 99 (2019) 489–510.

[49] Y. Han, L. Dai, Conducting polymers for flexible supercapacitors, *Macromolecular Chemistry and Physics*, 220 (2019) 1800355.

[50] M. Tomczykowa, M.E. Plonska-Brzezinska, Conducting polymers, hydrogels and their composites: Preparation, properties and bioapplications, *Polymers*, 11 (2019) 350.

[51] E.A. Kamoun, E-R.S. Kenawy, X. Chen, A review on polymeric hydrogel membranes for wound dressing applications: PVA-based hydrogel dressings, *Journal of Advanced Research*, 8 (2017) 217–233.

[52] J. Chen, Q. Peng, T. Thundat, H. Zeng, Stretchable, injectable, and self-healing conductive hydrogel enabled by multiple hydrogen bonding toward wearable electronics, *Chemistry of Materials*, 31 (2019) 4553–4563.

[53] B. Guo, L. Glavas, A-C. Albertsson, Biodegradable and electrically conducting polymers for biomedical applications, *Progress in Polymer Science*, 38 (2013) 1263–1286.

[54] F. Gao, W. Xie, Y. Miao, D. Wang, Z. Guo, A. Ghosal, Y. Li, Y. Wei, S-S. Feng, L. Zhao, H.M. Fan, Magnetic hydrogel with optimally adaptive functions for breast cancer recurrence prevention, *Advanced Healthcare Materials 8* (2019), 1900203.

[55] A. Vashist, A. Kaushik, R.D. Jayant, A. Vashist, A. Ghosal, M. Nair, Hydrogels: Stimuli responsive to on-demand drug delivery systems, in: A. Kaushik, R.D. Jayant, M. Nair (Eds.) *Advances in Personalized Nanotherapeutics*, Springer International Publishing, Cham, 2017, pp. 117–130.

[56] A. Vashist, A. Kaushik, A. Ghosal, J. Bala, R. Nikkhah-Moshaie, W.A. Wani, P. Manickam, M. Nair, Nanocomposite hydrogels: Advances in nanofillers used for nanomedicine, *Gels*, 4 (2018) 75.

[57] A. Mishra, A. Ghosal, Synthesis and applications of biopolymeric nanoparticles, in *Biopolymers and Nanocomposites for Biomedical and Pharmaceutical Applications*, Nova Science Publisher 51, 2017

[58] F. Zafar, A. Ghosal, E. Sharmin, R. Chaturvedi, N. Nishat, A review on cleaner production of polymeric and nanocomposite coatings based on waterborne polyurethane dispersions from seed oils. *Progress in Organic Coatings*. 131, (2019), 259–75.

[59] A. Ghosal, A. Vashist, S. Tiwari, E. Sharmin, S. Ahmad, J. Bhattacharya, Nanotechnology for therapeutics, in: *Advances in Personalized Nanotherapeutics*, Springer, 2017, pp. 25–40.

[60] A. Vashist, A. Kaushik, A. Vashist, V. Sagar, A. Ghosal, Y. Gupta, S. Ahmad, M. Nair, Advances in carbon nanotubes—hydrogel hybrids in nanomedicine for therapeutics, *Advanced Healthcare Materials*, 7 (2018) 1701213.

[61] D. Mawad, E. Stewart, D.L. Officer, T. Romeo, P. Wagner, K. Wagner, G.G. Wallace, A single component conducting polymer hydrogel as a scaffold for tissue engineering, *Advanced Functional Materials*, 22 (2012) 2692–2699.

[62] M. Gizdavic-Nikolaidis, S. Ray, J. Bennett, S. Swift, G. Bowmaker, A. Easteal, Electrospun poly (aniline-co-ethyl 3-aminobenzoate)/poly (lactic acid) nanofibers and their potential in biomedical applications, *Journal of Polymer Science Part A: Polymer Chemistry*, 49 (2011) 4902–4910.

[63] M. Shahadat, M.Z. Khan, P.F. Rupani, A. Embrandiri, S. Sultana, S.Z. Ahammad, S.W. Ali, T. Sreekrishnan, A critical review on the prospect of polyaniline-grafted biodegradable nanocomposite, *Advances in Colloid and Interface Science*, 249 (2017) 2–16.

[64] P. Srisuk, F.V. Berti, L.P. da Silva, A.P. Marques, R.L. Reis, V.M. Correlo, Electroactive gellan gum/polyaniline spongy-like hydrogels, *ACS Biomaterials Science & Engineering*, 4 (2018) 1779–1787.

4 Smart Hydrogels and Their Responsiveness

Eijaz Ahmed Bhat, Nasreena Sajjad, Wasifa Noor, Ifrah Manzoor, and Durdana Shah

CONTENTS

4.1 INTRODUCTION

The area of research regarding reactive materials has been improved by the advancement of hydrogels as useful biomaterials [1]. Primarily for contact lenses and tissue scaffolds, hydrogels were established for biomedical use. At the end of the 19th century, hydrogels were initially reported as colloidal gels from inorganic salt. Presently, hydrogel is described as networks of hydrophilic polymers arranged in a three-dimensional structure. These complexes have the capability to bulge and imbibe high quantities of biological liquids or water without scrapping their structure. The polymer chains, for example, amide, carboxyl, amino, and hydroxyl groups, have hydrophilic compounds linked to them which are responsible for their capability to absorb fluids and have the capability to get ionized in the existence of water. Moreover, elasticity and mechanical tolerance, which are crucial characteristics to be regarded when establishing delivery systems, can be enhanced by changing their physical characteristics—for example, mechanical strength, swelling, and surface characteristics through physicochemical reactions. The most frequent application terms related to hydrogels are 'ocular lens', 'wound healing' [2], 'super-absorbents', 'tissue engineering', 'tissue scaffolds', 'cell immobilization', and 'drug delivery systems' [3]. The increased growth in the number of publications has been documented in the Science Direct database comprising hydrogels with these keywords. Even though this preponderance can be seen for all earlier described subjects, tissue engineering and drug delivery stand out as they constitute the most of the publications. Remarkably, a similar increase in studies regarding tissue scaffolds, tissue engineering, wound healing, and drug delivery have been reported. The increase in the count of publications containing the term 'hydrogels' was noted since 2000 [4]. Concurrently, researchers and several industry segments are getting consideration towards hydrogels as for their use as applicative substances [5]. They display swelling/deswelling characteristics connected with the accessibility of water. In the chemical, physical, and biological research, hydrogels of these kinds are associated with their exclusive characteristics that can be related to environmental determinants. Kuhn and co-workers in 1948 established the term 'smart' even though the primary research related to hydrogels occurred in 1894 [6]. The most contemporary nomenclature is able to establish distinct triggers (stimuli) to create alterations in organization and function and, thus, acquired significance. The primary publication established was on molecules of poly(acrylic acid) polymer that are able to sustain structural changes in accordance with the cell culture media, pH [7]. However, publications established specific profiles for distinct networks of polymers inclusive of the new smart hydrogels. Drug delivery is able to recognize the persisting stimuli responsiveness via functional, morphological, or structural alterations initiating the discharge of trapped drugs in a coordinated way [8].

There are several measures by which smart hydrogels may be categorized. Degradability, origin (natural or synthetic), and cross-linking methods for self-assembly are among the set of measures that have been utilized to categorize these hydrogels. Chemically covalent bound linking of polymer chains leading to persistent connections gives rise to cross-linked networks within hydrogels [9]. On the contrary, supramolecular forces (non-covalent) are responsible for physically cross-linked structures, resulting in rapid and alterable systems [10]. Other classifications are based on the type of stimuli responsiveness such as physical or chemical stimuli. The pioneer kinds of physical responses consist of pressure, temperature, light, and magnetic or electric fields. Biochemical or chemical stimulants consist of pH, ionic strength, and ions [11]. Biological stimuli indicate response to the molecular processes—for example, catalytic reactions and identification of receptors present on the molecules. In addition, these networks may be formulated to act on single or several stimuli indexes [12]. This chapter concentrates on the fundamental ideas and reactive methods directed by changing the constituents that can impart helpful tools for formulating smart hydrogels in useful ways.

4.2 HYDROGELS AND RESPONSIVENESS

Hydrogels have consisted of networks of polymer with three-dimensional (3D) microstructures showing an upper hydration level and exhibiting similarity to natural tissue [2, 3]. 'Smart' hydrogels could alterably react to outer stimuli such as temperature, pH, pressure, electrical fields, light, solvent, ionic strength, etc. In the initial 1960s, they were one of the primary biomaterials prepared for clinical application by Otto Wichterle and Drahoslav Lim [13]. However, their promising use in several areas has drawn high attention in the past two decades. They may undergo phase transitions or sol-gel phase transitions due to change in surroundings, which can cause drug discharge, engineering of tissue, soft machines, etc. [14, 15]. Out of these uses, these 'intelligent' or smart polymers have acted as a crucial part in managing the place of drug release as well as time of delivery and, thus, have resulted in extraordinary development in drug release systems [16].

4.3 KEY TYPES OF RESPONSIVE SMART POLYMER HYDROGELS

Many kinds of smart hydrogels occur, such as those which respond to pH, temperature, ions, light, glucose, or electricity or are multi-responsive materials. Certain new, state-of-the-art instances of every hydrogel class as well as distinct kinds of smart hydrogels and their particular characteristics will be discussed in the following portion.

4.3.1 TEMPERATURE-RESPONSIVE HYDROGELS

In reaction to the environmental temperature, temperature-reactive smart hydrogels alter their structural characteristics. They include the often researched reactive networks possessing the high capability for several biomedical practices. Temperature-reactive hydrogels could be categorized as negatively temperature-sensitive lower critical solution temperature (LCST) and positively temperature-sensitive upper critical solution temperature (UCST) polymers [17, 18]. Unfavorably, thermosensitive hydrogels consist of an LCST and shrink when heated higher than the LCST. This kind of bulging action is called the inverse (or negative) temperature dependence. Inverse temperature-dependent hydrogels include polymer chains that either consist of slightly non-polar groups or a blend of polar and non-polar components. In this case, hydrophobic polymer chains would be present, and no dissolution in water whatsoever could occur. Increased dissolution occurs at decreased temperatures as creation of hydrogen bonds among polar components in the polymer chain and molecules of water overrules. As the temperature increases, the creation of hydrogen bonds decreases whereas interactivity between non-polar components increases significantly. As a consequence, the hydrogel contracts because of the interactions between interpolymer chains complementing the non-polar associations. Curiously, the LCST is reduced with the enhancing quantity of non-polar components existing in the polymer backbone [19]. Overall, LCST networks are chiefly concerning when focusing on managed drug delivery, specifically for proteins discharge [20, 21]. Copolymers consisting of (N-isopropylacrylamide) (PNIPAAm) are commonly practiced as LCST polymers. The decrease and increase in temperatures of PNIPAAm-based hydrogels exhibit an on/off drug discharge, respectively, allowing periodic and systematic on-demand drug delivery [22–24]. A positively thermosensitive hydrogel is distinguished by a UCST. If the temperature of cooling is less than the UCST, these hydrogels shrink. Positive temperature-determined bulging is exhibited by polymer systems comprising poly (acrylic acid) (PAA) and polyacrylamide (PAAm) [25]. Usually applied temperature-reactive materials are those made from poly (ethylene oxide)-b-poly(propylene oxide)-b poly (ethylene oxide) (Pluronics R, Tetronics R, poloxamer) [26, 27]. The solution of polymer, a running fluid at normal temperature and a gel at body temperature, are subjected to be Pluronic. Through integrating components reactive to temperature such as Pluronic F127 or PNIPAAm, receptivity to temperature responsiveness may be attained. Thus, thermosensitive cross-linking segments can be utilized for constructing temperature-sensitive hydrogels [28, 29]. During the preparation of thermosensitive hydrogels, fresh dimensions are adjoined when the thermosensitive cross-linking segments, similarly in PNIPAAm hydrogels, which are reactive to temperature, react with mobile cross-linking sites through the radical copolymerization with cyclic poly (ethylene glycol) (PEG) [17]. The hydrogel developed showed rapid volume bulging because of the enhanced polymer chains movement [30]. Highly branched amine-functionalized block copolymer of PEG-b-(L-lactide) is prepared by cross-linking of PEG and trifunctional PLLAs. The copolymers acquired exhibited temperature-reactive gelation from polymer solution concentration of ≥ 4 wt%. Curiously, by altering the copolymer amount and the molecular weight of the poly(L-lactide) blocks, the transition temperature can be calibrated. The hydrogels formed can be performed as an injectable agent, allowing development of in situ gel [31]. The hydrogel network was made of a 3-arm star copolymer utilizing a β-cyclodextrin (β-CD) core via consecutive reversible addition-fragmentation polymerization (RAFT) method. The β-CD xanthate was utilized as a segment of chain transfer. The star-tailored copolymer arms composed of polar poly (N, N-dimethylacrylamide) (PDMA) blocks and PNIPAAm blocks are reactive to temperature. The copolymer is soluble because each of the blocks is water dissolvable beneath the LCST of the PNIPAM component. Although, over the LCST, the blocks of PNIPAM get water unsolvable. Certain star-tailored topology and PNIPAAm chains get disintegrated thermally were generally accountable for the gelation.

4.3.2 pH-Responsive Smart Hydrogels

The pH-responsive hydrogels are produced from sensitive polymers susceptive to pH consisting of ionizable functional groups that either receive or give out protons in reaction with alterations in pH of environment [32–34]. The structural characteristics of these kinds of hydrogels changed at a pH higher and lower than fixed pH. A change of the hydrodynamic amount or the polymer chain configuration resulted due to the fast alteration in the pendant or backbone functionalities pertaining to pH.

Many polymers susceptible to pH are established on PAA (CarbopolR, carbomer) or by-products thereof containing poly(diethylaminoethyl methacrylate) (PDEAEMA) and poly(methacrylic acid) (PMAA) [35]. Furthermore, certain polymers including by-products of phosphoric acid have also been described [36, 37]. Polyelectrolytes are the term given to these polymers which consist of a high count of functional groups that are ionizable. The existence of ionizable groups in the polymer chains leads to enhanced hydrogel bulging in comparison to polymer hydrogels which are non-electrolyte. The bulging of polyelectrolyte hydrogels is primarily because of the electrostatic aversion taking place within charges existing on the polymer backbone, and the range of bulging is determined by elements decreasing electrostatic aversions.

For example, ionic strength, pH, and the kinds of counter ions existing in the system matter. In alkaline or neutral conditions, the pH-reactive character of hydrogels could be used for release of biomolecule. PAA, chitosan poly (dimethylamino-ethylmeth-acrylate) (PDMAEMA), and poly(ethylene imine) (PEI) are the polymers that consist of fundamental functional components containing primary, secondary, and tertiary amines which get ionized with the reduction in pH [38]. The pH reactiveness of PAA can be tuned through integration of acetal or ketal linkages within the backbone. On decreasing the pH, acetal and ketal linkages lead to the polymer disintegration of low molecular weight water-loving components. The pH-determined disintegration profile was indicated by polymers which were formed with a considerable rise in degree of hydrolysis when pH was decreased from 7.4 to 5.0 [39]. In a state of basic aqueous environment, a three-dimensional smart hydrogel reactive to pH is formed when the 1,3-benzene boronic acid forms a tetrahedral borate ester with the catechol end components of 4-arm PEG catechol [40]. Smart hydrogels reactive to pH were prepared by utilizing poly(lactic acid) (PLA), itaconic acid (IA) (P(LE-IA-MPEG)), and methoxyl poly(ethylene glycol) (MPEG) through polymerization of free radicals was induced by heating the lack of organic solvents. The consequences of the rate of pH on ratio of bulging were defined in buffers with pH varying from 1.2 to 6.8. The presence of carboxylic acids can be attributed to the existance of hydrogen bonds in the hydrogel at lower pH. As a consequence, motility and tranquility of the chain network are limited by the networks of these hydrogen bonds. When the pH is increased to 6.8, the carboxylic acid components get partly ionized, leading to the disintegration of the hydrogen bonds and the formation of electrostatic aversions within the chains of polymer, ultimately resulting in the bulging of hydrogel [41]. A triblock copolymer of smart hydrogel reactive to pH possessing pH-susceptible poly(2-(diisopropylamino) ethylmethacrylate) (PDPA) and biocompatible poly(2-(methacryloyloxy)-ethyl phosphorylcholine) (PMPC) have been reported. These hydrogels enabled calibrating the instinctive environment endured by myoblast cells of mouse. Through exact pH change, the flexibility of hydrogel can be controlled without influencing cell sustainability severely. The cells of myoblast showed noticeable development of stress fiber and straightening when hydrogel flexibility is enhanced. Appealingly, this idea could be used to investigate how cells change their morphology with regard to mechanical environment adjustment.

4.3.3 Light-Responsive Hydrogels

Smart hydrogels responsive to light are made up of networks of polymers consisting of groups that are responsive to light, for example, photochromic components. These hydrogels alter their physical and/or chemical characteristics, such as elasticity, form, viscosity, and rate of bulging, when illuminated with light. Integration of photochromic components into hydrogels have been achieved chemically (i.e., covalently) or physically (i.e., non-covalently) or through many other ways of cross-linking [42–44]. In the advanced display units, optical switches, and devices of ophthalmic drug release, hydrogels susceptible to light exhibit promising uses. The stimulus of light could be immediately applied and with significant precision is released in distinct doses, making these hydrogels susceptible to light. In engineering as well as biochemical areas, the enhancement of hydrogels susceptible to light is crucial because of their capability of immediate release when stimulus is administered. Hydrogels susceptible to light can be categorized into visible light-sensitive and UV-sensitive hydrogels [45]. A simple and direct way for the construction of PNIPAM/ graphene oxide (GO) nanocomposite hydrogels is by in situ γ-irradiation-facilitated polymerization of an aqueous solution of N-isopropylacrylamide and GO. The association of GO with PNIPAM brought about outstanding photothermal characteristics, where the reversible phase change in hydrogel was distantly influenced through subjection or non-subjection of laser. The outstanding photothermal susceptibility exhibited by nanocomposite hydrogels stimulated by light can broadly promise uses in biomaterials as well as microdevices. Exceptional characteristics applicable for the alterations in gels when required was showed by composite polypeptide (PC10P) hydrogel with gold nanorods. These gels went through immediate thermal changes through use of outer near-infrared (NIR) light, thereby imparting a method to control drug delivery [46]. When light is turned on, the components of azo are in the *cis* configuration, and the polymers of PAzo go through an alteration in structure to attain a coil form. As a consequence, the portion invaded by the PAzo chains rises, resulting in impetuous alteration in curvature and through the membrane 'curling' eruption of the huge vesicles. Griffin and co-workers produced smart hydrogels that are responsive to light, including photodegradable ortho-nitrobenzyl (o-NB) groups in the macromer backbone through redox polymerization. The apparent rate constants of the degradation were quantified using photorheology (at 370 nm, 10 mW/cm^2). The disintegration amount was enhanced excitingly when the count of aryl ethers on the o-NB group was reduced or altered by changing the functionality from primary to secondary at the benzylic site. The outcomes also showed that the hydrogels could be utilized to encase and discharge human mesenchymal stem cells (hMSCs) without impairing survivability of cells [47]. UCNPs, i.e., light-reactive hybrid up-conversion nanoparticles, were formed by Yan et al. (2012) from hydrogel systems, which characterized the first demonstration of how to apply the multi-photon effect of UCNPs to activate many structural changes in photophobic hydrogels. This study helps in the continuous-wave NIR light (980 nm) application, which later helps in the freedom of large biomolecules like enzymes and proteins entangled into the hydrogels and also helps in the induction of gel-sol transition.

4.3.4 ELECTRO-RESPONSIVE SMART HYDROGELS

Electrically responsive smart hydrogels are proficient in performing mechanical work which includes expansion, elongation, contraction, and bending under the effect of an electric field which depends on the shape and its position in accordance with the electrodes [48]. When a hydrogel is placed perpendicular and parallel to the electrodes, shrinkage and bending are observed respectively. Bending of hydrogel is widely used for the making of mechanical devices, including artificial muscles, valves, switches, soft actuators, and molecular machines [49]. Reversible shrinkage of hydrogels is studied mainly for drug delivery. An electric field as the external stimulus offers certain advantages such as precise control with regard to the current magnitude, the duration of the electric pulses, the interval between pulses, etc.

Evidence has been reported on the use of electric currents in the form of ionotophoresis and electroporation in the field of transdermal drug delivery. Electro-responsive hydrogels are constructed from the polymers which consist of comparatively high concentrations of ionizable groups, similar to the pH-responsive hydrogels. Synthetic and naturally (chondroitin sulfate, hyaluronic acid, and agarose) occurring polymers, separately as well as in combination, have been explored for this purpose. Synthetic polymers applied are mostly (meth)acrylate based. Overall, the polymers which can be conducting in nature can be called electrically responsive polymers. For example, polythiophene shows inflammation, dwindling, or twisting when an external electric field is applied. Electro-responsive hydrogels have become attractive amongst different other hydrogels because they have high usage in controlled drug delivery [50]. In an incompletely hydrolyzed polyacrylamide gel, an electro-responsive separation and contraction phase have been detected. They also deswell, which may be due to the electrophoretic pressure gradient [50]. Osada and Hasebe in 1985 observed the same effect for water-swollen poly(2-acrylamido-2-methyl-1-propanesulfonic acid) gel with 30% loss of absorbed water when the electric field is applied [51]. The use of chitosan gels as matrices can also assess electrically modulated drug delivery [52]. In electrification studies, release-time outlines for neutral, anionic, and cationic drugs from hydrated chitosan gels were examined as a function of time in reaction to different currents [53]. Similarly, chondroitin-4-sulfate hydrogels are potential matrices enabling electro-controlled peptide and protein delivery. 3D semi-interpenetrating networks were developed by PAA and fibrin as electro-responsive smart hydrogels from free radical polymerization [54]. Cross-linking between the two can be achieved by using initiators (ammonium persulfate, tetramethylethylenediamine) and an accelerator (N,N-methylenebisacrylamide). The electrical hydrogel stimulus ensured an enhanced penetration of cells and configuration inside the tissue, which can be useful in improving culture and seeding conditions for development of vascular grafts. Improvement in migration of cells and perfusion of cell through the culture medium during the scaffold after smearing a continuous stimulus pattern can be observed [54].

4.3.5 IONIC-RESPONSIVE CATIONIC POLYMERS

Ions play a critical role in most living processes. Thus, the application of polymeric hydrogels which are ion sensitive could intensely increase and improve their beneficial value [55–57]. Ionic responsiveness of polymers can be described as experiencing relatively rapid chemical and physical changes in reaction to minor outdoor changes in the concentration of ions. The concentration of ions in solvents is the crucial role in the exchanges among the final molecular conformation of polymeric chains. Ion-sensitive properties have been shown among P(DMAEMA-co-acrylic acid) copolymer, which forms a stable ionic complex with methylene blue and exhibits ion-sensitive drug release properties. The drug is freed from the polymer when copolymer hydrogel comes in contact with the isotonic sodium chloride solution [58]. The addition of NaCl in the solution gives rise to higher ionic strength, less repulsion, and more coiled conformation. PDMAEMA-g-PEG hydrogel nanoparticles are also expected to have ion-sensitive properties. The increase in ionic strength reduces the size of the cationic nanoparticles due to decrease in the osmotic pressure inside the polymeric nets. A constant increase in the ionic strength will break all the hydrogen bonds and result in accumulation of hydrogel nanoparticles [59, 60].

4.3.6 GLUCOSE-SENSITIVE HYDROGELS

Glucose-sensitive hydrogels are intelligent stimuli-responsive delivery systems using hydrogels that can release insulin and are a field of demanding research [61–63]. The development of self-regulated and/or modulated insulin delivery systems is one of the challenges in the controlled drug delivery area. The exact amount of insulin at the exact time of need has to be delivered, which requires a self-regulated insulin delivery system with glucose-sensing ability and an automatic shut-off mechanism. Several hydrogel systems with glucose sensors built into the system have already been developed for modulating insulin delivery. In response to a specific blood glucose level, pH-sensitive polymers containing immobilized insulin and glucose oxidase can swell, enabling insulin to release in a pulsatile fashion. The competitive binding of insulin or insulin and glucose to a fixed number of binding sites in concanavalin A (Con A) is another approach. Insulin is removed in response to glucose stimuli, thus functioning as a self-regulating insulin delivery system. In modulated insulin delivery, Con A has often been used. Insulin molecules are attached to a support or carrier through specific interactions in this type of system, which can be interrupted by glucose itself. D-glucose-sensitive hydrogel membranes were prepared based on cross-linking carboxymethyl dextran with the glucose-binding lectin Con A using carbodiimide chemistry [64]. Protein diffusion studies have revealed that the hydrogel permeability increases in response to changes in the D-glucose concentration of the external medium and causes competitive displacement of the cross-links based on affinity. By incorporating 3-phenylboronic acid, a tertiary amine, and dimethyl aminopropylacrylamide into a hydrogel matrix, the glucose-selective optical sensors are fabricated. The glucose-induced hydrogel contraction is responsible for the determination of glucose in solution. For glucose variations in ex vivo blood plasma was collected in the presence of ethylene diaminetetraacetic acid (EDTA) as anticoagulant, the sensor showed a very good response. A new comb type, glucose-responsive poly(NIPAM-co-AAPBA) grafted hydrogel, with rapid response to changes in blood glucose concentration at physiological temperature, was also developed by thermoresponsive poly (N-isopropylacrylamide) (PNIPAM) groups as actuators and phenylboronic acid (PBA) as glucose-sensing groups [65]. A smart glucose-responsive hydrogel was prepared by immobilizing the glucose/galactose binding protein (GBP) within an acrylamide hydrogel network [61]. A dynamic response to the presence of glucose and induced conformational change of *Escherichia coli*, glucose-binding protein trigger a mechanical action within a hydrogel network. Quantitative measurement to the glucose concentration was reported through demonstration of glucose-gated selective molecular transport. A series of glucose-sensitive hydrogels were synthesized by photopolymerization of glycidyl methacrylate (GMA)-modified dextran (Dex-G), ethylene glycol acrylate methacrylate (EGAMA)-modified concanavalin A (ConA–E), and poly(ethylene glycol) dimethacrylate (PEGDMA) [66]. It has also been noticed that hydrogels obtained from dextran and Con A have the ability to change in response to different glucose concentrations in the environment, owing to the reversible, specific lectin-saccharide-binding property [66]. The present literature studies have confirmed that the hydrogels showed good glucose-sensitive properties and biocompatibility.

4.3.7   MULTI-RESPONSIVE SMART HYDROGELS

Multi-responsive smart hydrogels show the response for two or more external stimuli, which provides the manipulation of a hydrogel system to get better targeting and efficacy in complex microenvironments or when used for other functions [67–69]. By conjugating the PAA to PEG via Michael addition polymerization, dual sensitivity was reported for a novel triblock copolymer of poly(amidoamine)-poly(ethylene glycol)-poly(amidoamine) (PAA-PEG-PAA) [70]. The PAA block works as a pH and temperature-sensitive block. The copolymer solution (12.5 wt%) was immediately transformed into a gel after injection into a rat. Apart from it the hydrogels also showed degradability and lack of cytotoxicity. Other reports of such hydrogels are also present in the literature.

4.4   SHORTCOMING IN SMART HYDROGELS

Smart hydrogels are polymeric systems with a three-dimensional network of cross-linked responsive polymer chains [71]. On the contribution of the conformational change of phase transition of the responsive polymeric chains in response to external chemical and/or physical stimuli, the smart hydrogels are able to change their volume, transparency, or other property. The smart hydrogels are developed with temperature-responsive, pH-responsive, ion-responsive, electro-responsive, light-responsive, glucose concentration–responsive, and other stimuli-responsive properties [72]. Because of the responsiveness and the capacity for abundant water or biological fluids, the smart hydrogels are often described as biological tissues such as cartilage and muscle. Thus, the smart hydrogels show significant potential for various applications, such as smart sensors/actuators, on/off switches, drug delivery vehicles, artificial muscles, tissue engineering scaffolds, and chemical-separation/bioseparation platforms [73–75]. The responsiveness and mechanical properties are critical parameters of the smart hydrogels. In the case-dependent applications such as smart actuators, artificial tissue, and soft robots, rapid responsiveness is desired for instantaneous and remarkable feedback after receiving environmental stimuli, while strong mechanical properties can tolerate large deformability under the external force. However, most of the smart hydrogels suffer from slow response speed and/or weak mechanical properties. The kinetics of swelling and deswelling in these hydrogels are typically governed by diffusion-limited transport of water molecules in the 3D polymeric network because of the dense skin layer of the hydrogel. The dense skin layer is usually formed during the fabrication process, as a common example, of free radical polymerization [76]. Furthermore, the responsive hydrogels also have poor mechanical properties because of the heterogeneous polymeric networks. In other words, when the hydrogels are synthesized by chain-growth polymerization with monomer and a certain amount of cross-linkers in an aqueous medium, the responsive hydrogels with highly heterogeneous structures are usually formed owing to different reactivity of the monomer and the cross-linking agent. During the network formation process, dense clusters are formed at the earlier stages of chain-growth polymerization and are connected by bridge polymeric chains at the following stages. However, after formation of the clusters, the polymerizing solution becomes more viscous, resulting in an asymmetrical distribution of clusters in the hydrogel. As a result, the bridge polymer length among the clusters is significantly diversified. Compared with the longer polymeric chains that require more energy to fracture, the shorter ones act as stress concentrators. When microcracks are formed at the short polymeric chains, macroscopic cracks can eventually be induced and propagated among the network. Thus, synthetic responsive hydrogels are notoriously weak due to their heterogeneous network. Many efforts have been devoted to improving the responsiveness and mechanical properties of hydrogels.

Several strategies have been developed with the aim of increasing the response dynamics by fabricating the responsive hydrogels with open-cell porous structures, comb-type structures, and microsphere- or micellar-containing nanocomposite structures [76, 77]. Creating hydrophilic regions for water pathways would aid the expulsion of water from the network during the collapse. Approaches have been developed to improve the mechanical properties of hydrogels by establishing double networks, topological networks, or nanocomposite networks cross-linked with exfoliated clay nanoparticles or microspheres. Thus, the nanocomposite responsive hydrogels exhibit improved responsiveness and mechanical properties which could simultaneously overcome the limitations of conventional chemically cross-linked hydrogels owing to nanocomposite network structures. In 2000, Liang and co-workers reported a type of thermosensitive poly(N-isopropylacrylamide) (PNIPAM)-clay nanocomposite hydrogels with enhanced temperature response. Later, Haraguchi extended the concept of nanocomposite hydrogel, which possessed a unique organic-inorganic network. Furthermore, other organic and inorganic nanomaterials have been utilized as building blocks or covalent cross-linkers to obtain responsive hydrogels with either rapid responsiveness and/or high mechanical properties (Haraguchi et al., 2011). Due to simultaneously improved responsiveness and mechanical properties, the nanocomposite responsive hydrogels have been considered to be significantly interesting and important for specific applications.

4.5 MECHANISMS FOR IMPROVING RESPONSIVENESS

In the traditional responsive hydrogels cross-linked only with small molecules, the dense skin layer formed during the chain-growth polymerization retards the diffusion of water molecules among the interior of the hydrogel network during the swelling-shrinking process, which leads to slow responsiveness. The improved responsiveness of nanocomposite smart hydrogels can be attributed to their nanostructure networks, including, but not limited to, three strategies. The first case is building a nanocomposite smart hydrogel network by chemically cross-linking responsive nanogels into the network structure. The responsive rate of the smart hydrogels is inversely proportional to the square of the small dimension of the hydrogel. The responsive nanogels are primarily shrinking to leave large amounts of voids and channels inside the nanocomposite hydrogel. At this stage, the porous structure of microsphere matrixes interconnects the water pathway, allowing the water to escape from the hydrogel matrixes. Using activated responsive nanogels as cross-linkers, the nanostructured smart responsive hydrogels are featured with fast response. Moreover, the polymeric chains bridging the nanogels are uniformly long. The bridging chains and dangling chains are freely mobilizable, resulting in a large equilibrium-swelling ratio. Second, doping other functional nanomaterials enables the construction of a diffusion passage or platform in the hydrogel matrix. For example, the electro-responsive property of the hydrogel is improved by adding conductive nanoparticles such as carbon nanotube, rGO, and so on. The hydrogel composed of polyelectrolyte can possess electro-responsive swelling/deswelling or bending/unbending behaviors. The deformation is driven by the osmotic pressure difference between inside and outside of the microgel, which is caused by the ionic concentration gradient in the hydrogel network along the direction of the electric field. Because of the charge groups that are restricted by the cross-linked networks in the hydrogel, only the mobile counterions can migrate toward the electrodes under electric field. Thus, the ion movements result in an ionic concentration gradient, leading to the osmotic pressure difference. When introducing the conductive nanoparticles in the hydrogel network, the functional nanomaterials provide conductive platforms for the promotion of ion movement among the hydrogel nanocomposite network under electric field. As a result, compared with the normal electro-responsive hydrogel without functional nanomaterials, the smart hydrogel with nanocomposite structure exhibits fast and significant response to electrical stimulus. Third, when the nanocomposite smart hydrogel is clay cross-linked with low effective cross-link density, the hydrogel shows a fast deswelling rate because the nanocomposite smart hydrogels cross-linked with clay's own structural homogeneity. With a lower content of clay, the mobility of responsive polymeric chains is considerably high. Thus, the water channels can be formed throughout the hydrogel due to the microenvironmental phase separation of the polymer. As a result, the shrinking proceeds quickly on a macroscopic scale, resulting from squeezing out the water from the internal hydrogel network. When increasing the clay content in the hydrogel network, the mobility of PNIPAM chains is gradually restricted due to the clay cross-linking. Therefore, the deswelling rate decreases on increasing the clay content, although the structural homogeneity is unchanged due to the homogeneous cross-linking.

4.6   CONCLUSIONS AND PERSPECTIVE

This chapter provided an overview of the progress that has been made to develop nanocomposite smart hydrogels and the strategies that have been adopted to improve the responsiveness and the mechanical properties of conventional hydrogels. Most of the conventional smart hydrogels suffer from slow response speed and/or weak mechanical properties. Several strategies have been developed with the aim of increasing the response dynamics by fabricating the responsive hydrogels with nanocomposite structures. Contrarily, other approaches have been developed to improve the mechanical properties of hydrogels, such as nanocomposite networks cross-linked with exfoliated clay nanoparticles or microspheres. The nanomaterials can also be used to act as simple fillers by blending them in the hydrogel matrix, resulting in the improvement of the mechanical properties of the nanocomposite hydrogels. By incorporating nanomaterials into the hydrogel networks, improvement in responsiveness and mechanical properties can be simultaneously achieved. Since responsiveness and mechanical properties are paramount for many applications, the nanocomposite smart hydrogels demonstrate potential applications such as in artificial muscle, soft robots, tissue engineering scaffolds, and many others. However, there still remain several important issues that must be addressed in the future. First, to date, only thermo-responsive, pH-responsive, electro-responsive, near-infrared-light-responsive nanocomposite hydrogels have been developed. Therefore, in order to improve the functionality of nanocomposite hydrogels, it is important that future efforts should focus on developing and investigating some other stimuli- or multi-responsive hydrogels. Second, the number of studies that have been carried out on nanocomposite smart hydrogels within the last two decades is quite limited. Therefore, in order to widen the application range of nanocomposite smart hydrogels, further improvement should be sought in terms of responsiveness, including responsive rate and degree, as well as mechanical properties, including Young's modulus, toughness, breaking strength, breaking strain, and so on. Third, future studies with the focus on the regulations of the interactions between nanomaterials and hydrogel polymeric chains are crucial. Fourth, since nanocomposite smart hydrogels can have potential applications in biomedical and biological areas, the biocompatibility verification of these nanocomposite materials is absolutely necessary.

REFERENCES

[1]   Huebsch, N., & Mooney, D. J. Inspiration and application in the evolution of biomaterials. *Nature*, **462**(7272), 426–432, 2009.
[2]   Cushing, M. C., & Anseth, K. S. Materials science: Hydrogel cell cultures. *Science*, **316**(5828), 1133–1134, 2007.
[3]   Merdan, T., Kopeček, J., & Kissel, T. Prospects for cationic polymers in gene and oligonucleotide therapy against cancer. *Advanced Drug Delivery Reviews*, **54**(5), 715–758, 2002.
[4]   Lee, S. C., Kwon, I. K., & Park, K. Hydrogels for delivery of bioactive agents: A historical perspective. *Advanced Drug Delivery Reviews*, **65**, 17–20, 2013.
[5]   Chu, L-Y., Xie, R., Ju, X-J., & Wang, W. *Smart hydrogel functional materials*. Springer-Verlag, Berlin, Heidelberg, 2013.
[6]   Kuhn, W. Reversible Dehnung und Kontraktion bei Änderung der Ionisation eines Netzwerks polyvalenter Fadenmolekülionen. *Experientia*, **5**, 318–319, 1949.
[7]   Richter, A. Hydrogel-based μTAS, in: Leondes, C. T. (ed.) *MEMS/NEMS handbook: Techniques and applications*. Springer, New York, pp. 141–171, 2006.
[8]   Zheng, H., Xing, L., Cao, Y., & Che, S. Coordination bonding based pH-responsive drug delivery systems. *Coordination Chemistry Reviews*, **257**, 1933–1944, 2013.
[9]   Buwalda, S. J., Boere, K. W., Dijkstra, P. J., Feijen, J., Vermonden, T., & Hennink, W. E. Hydrogels in a historical perspective: From simple networks to smart materials. *Journal of Controlled Release*, **190**, 254–273, 2014.
[10] Amin, M. C. I. M., Ahmad, N., Pandey, M., Abeer, M. M., & Mohamad, N. Recent advances in the role of supramolecular hydrogels in drug delivery. *Expert Opinion on Drug Delivery*, **12**, 1149–1161, 2015.

[11] Samchenko, Y., Ulberg, Z., & Korotych, O. Multipurpose smart hydrogel systems. *Advances in Colloid and Interface Science*, **168**, 247–262, 2011.

[12] Samal, S. K., Dash, M., Dubruel, P., & Van Vlierberghe, S. Smart polymer hydrogels: Properties, synthesis and applications, in: De Armas, M. R. A. & Román, J. S. (eds.) *Smart polymers and their applications.* Woodhead Publishing, Cambridge, pp. 237–270, 2014.

[13] Kopecek, J. Hydrogels: From soft contact lenses and implants to self-assembled nano-materials. *Journal of Polymer Science Part A: Polymer Chemistry*, **47**(22), 5929–5946, 2009.

[14] Bajpai, A. K., Shukla, S. K., Bhanu, S., & Kankane, S. Responsive polymers in con-trolled drug delivery. *Progress in Polymer Science*, **33**(11), 1088–1118, 2008.

[15] Ilg, P. Stimuli-responsive hydrogels cross-linked by magnetic nanoparticles. *Soft Matter*, **9**(13), 3465, 2013.

[16] Peppas, N. A., Hilt, J. Z., Khademhosseini, A., & Langer, R. Hydrogels in biology and medicine: From molecular principles to bionanotechnology. *Advanced Materials*, **18**(11), 1345–1360, 2006.

[17] Ishida, K., Uno, T., Itoh, T., & Kubo, M. Synthesis and property of temperature-respon-sive hydrogel with movable cross-linking points. *Macromolecules*, **45**, 6136–6142, 2012.

[18] Qiu, Y., & Park, K. Environment-sensitive hydrogels for drug delivery. *Advanced Drug Delivery Reviews*, **53**, 321–339, 2001.

[19] Huber, S., Hutter, N., & Jordan, R. Effect of end group polarity upon the lower critical solution temperature of poly(2-isopropyl-2-oxazoline). *Colloid and Polymer Science*, **286**, 1653–1661, 2008.

[20] Bromberg, L. E., & Ron, E. S. Temperature-responsive gels and thermogelling poly-mer matrices for protein and peptide delivery. *Advanced Drug Delivery Reviews*, **31**, 197–221, 1998.

[21] Hassouneh, W., Macewan, S. R., & Chilkoti, A. Chapter nine—fusions of elastin-like polypeptides to pharmaceutical proteins, in: Wittrup, K. D. & Gregory, L. V. (eds.) *Methods in enzymology.* Academic Press, Elsevier B. V. Cambridge, 2012.

[22] Prabaharan, M., & Mano, J. F. Stimuli-responsive hydrogels based on polysaccharides incorporated with thermo-responsive polymers as novel biomaterials. *Macromolecular Bioscience*, **6**, 991–1008, 2006.

[23] Satarkar, N. S., Biswal, D., & Hilt, J. Z. Hydrogel nanocomposites: A review of applica-tions as remote controlled biomaterials. *Soft Matter*, **6**, 2364–2371, 2010.

[24] Trongsatitkul, T., & Budhlall, B. M. Microgels or microcapsules? Role of morphology on the release kinetics of thermoresponsive PNIPAm-co-PEGMa hydrogels. *Polymer Chemistry*, **4**, 1502–1516, 2013.

[25] Ward, M. A., & Georgiou, T. K. Thermoresponsive polymers for biomedical applica-tions. *Polymers*, **3**, 1215–1242, 2011.

[26] Bromberg, L. Synthesis and self-assembly of poly(ethylene oxide)-bpoly(propylene oxide)-b-poly(ethylene oxide)-g-poly(acrylic acid) gels. *Industrial and Engineering Chemistry Research*, 2437–2444, 2001.

[27] Fernandez-Tarrio, M., Yañez, F., Immesoete, K., Alvarez-Lorenzo, C., & Concheiro, A. Pluronic and tetronic copolymers with polyglycolyzed oils as selfemulsifying drug delivery systems. *AAPS PharmSciTech*, **9**, 471–479, 2008.

[28] Hamcerencu, M., Desbrieres, J., Popa, M., & Riess, G. R. Stimuli-sensitive xanthan derivatives/N-isopropylacrylamide hydrogels: Influence of cross-linking agent on interpenetrating polymer network properties. *Biomacromolecules*, **10**, 1911–1922, 2009.

[29] Wang, C., Stewart, R. J., & Kopecek, J. Hybrid hydrogels assembled from synthetic polymers and coiled-coil protein domains. *Nature*, **397**, 417–420, 1999.

[30] Velthoen, I. W., VAN Beek, J., Dijkstra, P. J., & Feijen, J. Thermo-responsive hydrogels based on highly branched poly(ethylene glycol)—poly(l-lactide) copolymers. *Reactive and Functional Polymers*, **71**, 245–253, 2011.

[31] Zhang, H., Yan, Q., Kang, Y., Zhou, L., Zhou, H., Yuan, J., & Wu, S. Fabrication of thermo-responsive hydrogels from star-shaped copolymer with a biocompatible β -cyclodextrin core. *Polymer*, **53**, 3719–3725, 2012.

[32] Dou, X-Q., Yang, X-M., Li, P., Zhang, Z-G., Schonherr, H., Zhang, D., & Feng, C-L. Novel pH responsive hydrogels for controlled cell adhesion and triggered surface detachment. *Soft Matter*, **8**, 9539–9544, 2012.

[33] Krogsgaard, M., Behrens, M. A., Pedersen, J. S., & Birkedal, H. Self-healing mussel-inspired multi-pH-responsive hydrogels. *Biomacromolecules*, **14**, 297–301, 2013.

[34] Schoener, C. A., Hutson, H. N., & Peppas, N. A. pH-responsive hydrogels with dispersed hydrophobic nanoparticles for the delivery of hydrophobic therapeutic agents. *Polymer International*, **61**, 874–879, 2012.

[35] Soppimath, K. S., Aminabhavi, T. M., Dave, A. M., Kumbar, S. G., & Rudzinski, W. E. Stimulus-responsive 'smart' hydrogels as novel drug delivery systems. *Drug Development and Industrial Pharmacy*, **28**, 957–974, 2002.

[36] Miyata, T., Nakamae, K., Hoffman, A. S., & Kanzaki, Y. Stimuli-sensitivities of hydrogels containing phosphate groups. *Macromolecular Chemistry and Physics*, **195**, 1111–1120, 1994.

[37] Nakamae, K., Miyata, T., & Hoffman, A. S. Swelling behavior of hydrogels containing phosphate groups. *Die Makromolekulare Chemie*, **193**, 983–990, 1992.

[38] Jain, R., Standley, S. M., & Fréchet, J. M. J. Synthesis and degradation of pH sensitive linear poly(amidoamine)s. *Macromolecules*, **40**, 452–457, 2007.

[39] He, L., Fullenkamp, D. E., Rivera, J. G., & Messersmith, P. B. pH responsive self-healing hydrogels formed by boronate-catechol complexation. *Chemical Communications*, **47**, 7497–7499, 2011.

[40] Wang, L., Liu, M., Gao, C., Ma, L., & Cui, D. A pH-, thermo-, and glucose-, triple-responsive hydrogels: Synthesis and controlled drug delivery. *Reactive and Functional Polymers*, **70**, 159–167, 2010.

[41] Yoshikawa, H. Y., Rossetti, F. F., Kaufmann, S., Kaindl, T., Madsen, J., Engel, U., Lewis, A. L., Armes, S. P., & Tanaka, M. Quantitative evaluation of mechanosensing of cells on dynamically tunable hydrogels. *Journal of the American Chemical Society*, **133**, 1367–1374, 2011.

[42] Alvarez-Lorenzo, C., Bromberg, L., & Concheiro, A. Light-sensitive intelligent drug delivery systems. *Photochemistry and Photobiology*, **85**, 848–860, 2009.

[43] Yan, B., Boyer, J-C., Habault, D., Branda, N. R., & Zhao, Y. Near infrared light triggered release of biomacromolecules from hydrogels loaded with upconversion nanoparticles. *Journal of the American Chemical Society*, **134**, 16558–16561, 2012.

[44] Zhao, Y-L., & Stoddart, J. F. Azobenzene-based light-responsive hydrogel system. *Langmuir*, **25**, 8442–8446, 2009.

[45] Zhu, C-H., Lu, Y., Peng, J., Chen, J-F., & Yu, S-H. Photothermally sensitive poly(N-isopropylacrylamide)/graphene oxide nanocomposite hydrogels as remote light-controlled liquid microvalves. *Advanced Functional Materials*, **22**, 4017–4022, 2012.

[46] Mabrouk, E., Cuvelier, D., Brochard-Wyart, F., Nassoy, P., & Li, M-H. Bursting of sensitive polymersomes induced by curling. *Proceedings of the National Academy of Sciences*, **106**, 7294–7298, 2009.

[47] Griffin, D. R., & Kasko, A. M. Photodegradable macromers and hydrogels for live cell encapsulation and release. *Journal of the American Chemical Society*, **134**, 13103–13107, 2012.

[48] Murdan, S. Electro-responsive drug delivery from hydrogels. *Journal of Controlled Release*, **92**, 1–17, 2003.

[49] Messing, R., & Schmidt, A. M. Perspectives for the mechanical manipulation of hybrid hydrogels. *Polymer Chemistry*, **2**, 18–32, 2011.

[50] Tanaka, T., Nishio, I., Sun, S-T., & Ueno-Nishio, S. Collapse of gels in an electric field. *Science*, **218**, 467–469, 1982.

[51] Osada, Y., & Hasebe, M. Electrically activated mechanochemical devices using poly-electrolyte gels. *Chemistry Letters*, **14**, 1285–1288, 1985.

[52] Ramanathan, S., & Block, L. H. The use of chitosan gels as matrices for electrically-modulated drug delivery. *Journal of Controlled Release*, **70**, 109–123, 2001.

[53] Jensen, M., Birch Hansen, P., Murdan, S., Frokjaer, S., & Florence, A. T. Loading into and electro-stimulated release of peptides and proteins from chondroitin 4-sulphate hydrogels. *European Journal of Pharmaceutical Sciences*, **15**, 139–148, 2002.

[54] Rahimi, N., Molin, D. G., Cleij, T. J., Van Zandvoort, M. A., & Post, M. J. Electrosensitive polyacrylic acid/fibrin hydrogel facilitates cell seeding and alignment. *Biomacromolecules*, **13**, 1448–1457, 2012.

[55] Chen, X., Li, W., Zhong, W., Lu, Y., & Yu, T. pH sensitivity and ion sensitivity of hydrogels based on complex-forming chitosan/silk fibroin interpenetrating polymer network. *Journal of Applied Polymer Science*, **65**, 2257–2262, 1997.

[56] Rasool, N., Yasin, T., Heng, J. Y. Y., & Akhter, Z. Synthesis and characterization of novel pH-, ionic strength and temperature- sensitive hydrogel for insulin delivery. *Polymer*, **51**, 1687–1693, 2010.

[57] Zhao, B., & Moore, J. S. Fast pH- and ionic strength-responsive hydrogels in micro-channels. *Langmuir*, **17**, 4758–4763, 2001.

[58] Sutani, K., Kaetsu, I., Uchida, K., & Matsubara, Y. Stimulus responsive drug release from polymer gel: Controlled release of ionic drug from polyampholyte gel. *Radiation Physics and Chemistry*, **64**, 331–336, 2002.

[59] Deng, L., Zhai, Y., Lin, X., Jin, F., He, X., & Dong, A. Investigation on properties of re-dispersible cationic hydrogel nanoparticles. *European Polymer Journal*, **44**, 978–986, 2008.

[60] Liu, X-W., Zhu, S., Wu, S-R., Wang, P., & Han, G-Z. Response behavior of ion-sensitive hydrogel based on crown ether. *Colloids and Surfaces A: Physicochemical and Engineering Aspects*, **417**, 140–145, 2013.

[61] Ehrick, J. D., Luckett, M. R., Khatwani, S., Wei, Y., Deo, S. K., Bachas, L. G., & Daunert, S. Glucose responsive hydrogel networks based on protein recognition. *Macromolecular Bioscience*, 864–868, 2009.

[62] Kim, J. J., & Park, K. Modulated insulin delivery from glucose-sensitive hydrogel dosage forms. *Journal of Controlled Release*, **77**, 39–47, 2001.

[63] Traitel, T., Cohen, Y., & Kost, J. Characterization of glucose-sensitive insulin release systems in simulated in vivo conditions. *Biomaterials*, **21**, 1679–1687, 2000.

[64] Zhang, R., Tang, M., Bowyer, A., Eisenthal, R., & Hubble, J. Synthesis and character-ization of a d-glucose sensitive hydrogel based on CM-dextran and concanavalin A. *Reactive and Functional Polymers*, **66**, 757–767, 2006.

[65] Zhang, S-B., Chu, L-Y., Xu, D., Zhang, J., Ju, X-J., & Xie, R. Poly(Nisopropylacrylamide)-based comb-type grafted hydrogel with rapid response to blood glucose concentration change at physiological temperature. *Polymers for Advanced Technologies*, **19**, 937–943, 2008.

[66] Yin, R., Wang, K., Han, J., & Nie, J. Photo-crosslinked glucose-sensitive hydrogels based on methacrylate modified dextran—concanavalin A and PEG dimethacrylate. *Carbohydrate Polymers*, **82**, 412–418, 2010.

[67] Dumitriu, R. P., Mitchell, G. R., & Vasile, C. Multi-responsive hydrogels based on N-isopropylacrylamide and sodium alginate. *Polymer International*, **60**, 222–233, 2011.

[68] Guenther, M., Kuckling, D., Corten, C., Gerlach, G., Sorber, J., Suchaneck, G., & Arndt, K. F. Chemical sensors based on multiresponsive block copolymer hydrogels. *Sensors and Actuators B: Chemical*, **126**, 97–106, 2007.

[69] Zhang, Y., Tao, L., Li, S., & Wei, Y. Synthesis of multiresponsive and dynamic chitosan-based hydrogels for controlled release of bioactive molecules. *Biomacromolecules*, **12**, 2894–2901, 2011.

[70] Nguyen, M. K., Park, D. K., & Lee, D. S. Injectable poly(amidoamine)- poly(ethylene glycol)-poly(amidoamine) triblock copolymer hydrogel with dual sensitivities: pH and temperature. *Biomacromolecules*, **10**, 728–731, 2009.

[71] Xia, L-W. *et al.* Nano-structured smart hydrogels with rapid response and high elasticity. *Nature Communications*, **4**, 2226, 2013.

[72] Yoshida, R., Uchida, K., Kaneko, Y., Sakai, K., Kikuchi, A., Sakurai, Y., & Okano, T. Comb-type grafted hydrogels with rapid deswelling response to temperature changes. *Nature*, **374**, 240, 1995.

[73] Stuart, M. A. C., Huck, W. T. S., Genzer, J., Müller, M., Ober, C., Stamm, M., Sukhorukov, G. B., Szleifer, I., Tsukruk, V. V., Urban, M., Winnik, F., Zauscher, S., Luzinov, I., & Minko, S. Emerging applications of stimuli-responsive polymer materials. *Nature Materials*, **9**, 101, 2010.

[74] Sidorenko, A., Krupenkin, T., Taylor, A., Fratzl, P., & Aizenberg, J. Reversible switching of hydrogel-actuated nanostructures into complex micropatterns. *Science*, **315**, 487, 2007.

[75] Nagase, K., Kobayashi, J., & Okano, T. Temperature-responsive intelligent interfaces for biomolecular separation and cell sheet engineering. *Journal of the Royal Society Interface*, **6**, S293, 2009.

[76] Zhang, X. Z., Xu, X. D., Cheng, S. X., & Zhuo, R. X. Strategies to improve the response rate of thermosensitive PNIPAAm hydrogels. *Soft Matter*, **4**, 385, 2008.

[77] Mou, C. L., Ju, X. J., Zhang, L., Xie, R. Wang, W., Deng, N. N., Wei, J., Chen, Q., & Chu, L. Y. Monodisperse and fast-responsive poly(N-isopropylacrylamide) microgels with open-celled porous structure. *Langmuir*. **30**, 1455, 2014.

5 Hydrogel for Sensing Applications

Tamal Sarkar, Tarun Kumar Dhiman and Partima R. Solanki

CONTENTS

5.1 INTRODUCTION

A hydrophilic three-dimensional (3D) cross-linked network swollen with water is referred to as a hydrogel. In another way, hydrogel can be defined as polymeric material that shows a capability to swell and retain a considerable amount of water inside its network but without dissolving in water [1]. Hydrogels can swell up to 99% (v/v) water of their weight without dissolution [2–4]. Hydrogels have gained significant attention from researchers over the last 50 years due to their extensive range of biomedical application in biosensing, tissue engineering, and drug delivery [5–7]. The large water body containing capability of hydrogel arises from the hydrophilic functional group attached to the monomer while their repellence to dissolution rises from the cross-link formation among polymer chains. The mostly inert nature and hydrophilicity of hydrogels are beneficial for minimizing the non-specific binding with cells and proteins which make hydrogels suitable candidates for several biomedical applications [8, 9]. By incorporating functional groups, hydrogels can be reactive to physical, chemical, and biochemical stimuli [10–13]. These stimuli produce reversible changes in swelling [14] and changes in refractive index (hydrogel microlenses) [15], causing gelation (for small molecule hydrogel) [16] and optical changes (e.g., fluorescence) [17]. In this chapter, classification, swelling mechanisms, and sensing applications of hydrogels have been reviewed.

5.2 CLASSIFICATION OF HYDROGELS

Different classifications based on various properties of hydrogels are charted here in Figure 5.1.

5.2.1 BASED ON THE NATURE OF CROSS-LINKING

Depending upon the nature of cross-linking, hydrogels are classified into two classes:

(i) *Chemically cross-linked hydrogels* form through covalent bonds. These hydrogels dissolve in water only after the breaking of covalent bonding [18, 19].

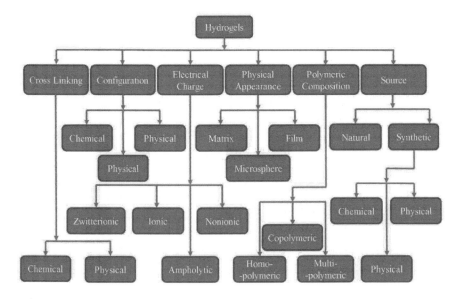

FIGURE 5.1   Classification of hydrogels based on properties.

(ii) *Physically cross-linked hydrogels* form through dynamic cross-linking of natural or synthetic building blocks. These hydrogels are formed via non-covalent interaction such as hydrogen bonding, hydrophobic interaction, and electrostatic interaction [20, 21].

5.2.2 BASED ON THE CONFIGURATION

Hydrogels can also be classified on the basis of the physical structure and the chemical nature as follows:

(i) *Amorphous hydrogels* are those which do not have long crystalline order of macromolecule chains. These hydrogels are colorless and transparent viscous gel containing polymer, glycerol, and water and are mainly used for wound dressing. Amorphous hydrogels create a moist wound environment without causing tissue maceration when in contact with a wound.

(ii) *Crystalline hydrogels* have very long-range crystalline order of macromolecule chains and are characterized by their crystalline nature.

(iii) *Semi-crystalline hydrogels* have short-range crystalline order. These can be considered as a mix of both crystalline and amorphous hydrogels. These have partial alignment of macromolecule chains.

5.2.3 BASED ON NETWORK ELECTRICAL CHARGE

Hydrogels can also be classified based on the presence or absence of the electrical charge localized on the cross-linked chains as follows:

(i) *Nonionic hydrogels* have neutral charge over them.

(ii) *Ionic hydrogels* polymers can have either cationic or anionic charge over them.

(iii) *Ampholytic hydrogels* have both the acidic or basic group attached in their structure.

(iv) *Zwitterionic hydrogels* contain both cations and anions simultaneously in there structure.

5.2.4 BASED ON PHYSICAL APPEARANCE

Depending upon the polymerization technique involved, hydrogels can be categorized as matrix, microsphere, or films.

5.2.5 BASED ON THE POLYMERIC COMPOSITION

(i) *Homopolymeric hydrogels* are derivative of single monomer. Depending upon the monomer and polymerization technique, homopolymers may possess cross-linked skeletal structure.

(ii) *Copolymeric hydrogels* consist of two or more different monomers, with one of them being hydrophilic in nature, organized at random or alternating configuration down the chain of polymeric network.

(iii) *Multipolymeric interpenetrating polymeric hydrogels* (IPN) are those in which two independent synthetic and/or natural polymers cross-link to form a polymeric network. Semi-IPN hydrogels are formed when one component is a cross-linked polymer and the other is a non-cross-linked polymer [22].

5.2.6 BASED ON THE SOURCE

Hydrogels are of two types based on their origins in natural or synthetic polymer.

5.2.6.1 Natural Hydrogel

Natural polymers are commonly biocompatible and biodegradable. Two major naturally occurring polymers are proteins (gelatin, collagen, and lysozyme) and polysaccharides (chitosan, alginate, and hyaluronic acid).

5.2.6.2 Synthetic Hydrogel

Synthetic hydrogels have a long life, high gel strength, and, of course, the capacity for a large amount of water absorption as compared to natural hydrogels. Properties of the synthetic polymer can be tuned in molecular scale to get desirable structure, functionality and degradability, chemical response, mechanical strength, and biological response to external stimuli. Derivatives of poly(hydroxyethyl methacrylate) (PHEMA), poly(vinyl alcohol) (PVA), and poly(ethylene glycol) (PEG) can be a neutral synthetic polymer. In many cases, PEG hydrogels have been used for biomedical application because they are non-immunogenic, non-toxic, and called 'stealth material' due to their inertness to most biological elements such as proteins [4, 23]. PEG hydrogels have been widely used through covalent bonding, adsorption, hydrogen, and ionic bonding to provide biocompatibility and surface protein resistance [4, 24]. PHEMA has also been extensively applied in biomedical applications such as drug delivery [25] and contact lenses [26]. The primary characteristics of PHEMA involve its optical transparency, mechanical properties, and stability in water. Physically cross-linked PVA has several biomedical applications due to its biodegradability [27–29]. Cross-linking in PVA can be achieved by the chemical, physical, or irradiative mechanism. Based on the response, synthetic hydrogels can be divided into three types.

5.2.6.2.1 Stimuli-Responsive Hydrogel

By tailoring the molecular structure of the polymer, environmentally responsive hydrogels can be synthesized to respond to external stimuli (e.g., pH, pI, and temperature) in an intelligent and programmed manner [30]. Recently, researchers have extensively studied the fabrication of environmentally responsive hydrogel sensitive to pH, temperature, and specific analytes.

The functionality of groups presents in the chain, branches, and cross-links are the chemical structural parameters that influence the response mechanism of the hydrogel. In networks containing weakly acidic or basic pendant groups, ionization starts after water sorption depending on the ionic composition and solution pH. The hydrogel behaves as a semipermeable membrane which balances osmotic pressure between the hydrogel and the surrounding solution through ion exchange. The equilibrium degree of swell increases for ionic gel, containing basic group as the pH of the surrounding solution decreases. The degree of swell increases as the pH of the solution increases for the acid group–containing ionic gel. Ionic content, nature of the polymer, and ionization equilibrium consideration are the main factors that influence the swelling of ionic hydrogels [31, 32]. Some well-studied ionic polymers are poly(methacrylate acid), poly(acrylic acid), etc.

Temperature-sensitive hydrogels are based on poly(N-isopropylacrylamide) (PNIPAAm) and its derivatives. These hydrogels go through a reversible phase transition when the temperature of the surrounding environment is changed. When the temperature is raised to a lower critical solution temperature (LCST), phase separation of the polymer occurs. PNIPAAm has LCST at around 33°C. Thermo-sensitive hydrogels have been applied widely in drug delivery and tissue engineering [33, 34].

5.2.6.2.2 Bioresponsive Hydrogel

Synthetic hydrogels can be integrated with biological entities to create bioresponsive hydrogels. Synthetic hydrogels synergistically unite biological mechanisms, such as specificity of binding, high accuracy, and high affinity with tunable hydrogel properties. Bioresponsive hydrogels can be prepared by incorporating bioactive molecules into the polymer network by physical or chemical entrapment [35]. Enzymes (e.g., glucose oxidase) have been incorporated into the network structure of pH-sensitive cationic hydrogel for glucose sensing [36]. Genetically engineered proteins-tailored hydrogels have been combined for potential drug delivery [37]. Hydrogels (e.g., PEG, alginate) have been modified with peptides derived from natural proteins to enhance cellular adhesion [38]. Hydrogels have also been modified with a degradable linker to utilize the degradation property [39]. The growth factor of a hydrogel (e.g., PEG) can also be modified by incorporating growth factors (e.g., TGF-β) into the network to control muscle cell functions [40]. Furthermore, hydrogels have been synthesized from genetically engineered polypeptides. Self-assembly of peptides was employed to synthesize hydrogel [41].

5.2.6.2.3 Imprinted Hydrogel

For many applications, the molecular recognition properties of hydrogels can be controlled via various biological analytes and physiological processes. For molecular recognition, structure and chemical functionality of the polymer can be precisely controlled in a 3D configuration. Template-mediated polymerization (e.g., molecular imprinting) techniques can be used to prepare polymers which can bind to template molecules with high accuracy [42]. These imprinted hydrogels have been applied for controlled drug delivery systems [43, 44].

5.3 THEORY OF SWELLING

The applicability of hydrogels as biomedical materials and their performances in the biomedical field rely to a large extent on their bulk structure. The fundamental parameters used to describe a network structure are as follows:

(i) The polymer volume fraction in the swollen state of hydrogel ($v_{2,s}$), $v_{2,s}$ is a quantification of the amount of water soaked and retained by the hydrogel.

(ii) Molecular weight of the polymer chain fraction between two consecutive cross-linked junctions $\overline{M_C}$, physical or chemical), which is a measure of the degree of cross-linking; only the verage value of the $\overline{M_C}$ can be calculated due to the random nature of polymerization.

(iii) Corresponding average mesh size (distance between two consecutive cross-linking points) (ζ), which is a measure of the gap between two macromolecular polymeric chains. These parameters can be determined by equilibrium-swelling theory or rubber-elasticity theory.

Hydrophilicity of a polymer produces an osmotic pressure within the hydrogel when exposed to water [45]. Swelling of the hydrogel is a three-step process: (i) water molecules diffuse through the matrix, (ii) polymer chains relax via hydration, and (iii) extension of polymer network via relaxation [46, 47]. The maximum amount of water which can be absorbed by the hydrogel is defined by the equilibrium of osmotic pressure and retractive forces of the polymer network. Flory-Rehner theory (equilibrium-swelling theory) can give a theoretical description of swelling of hydrogels which do not contain ionic moieties [48]. The theory states that if a cross-linked polymeric gel is immersed in a fluid and allowed to achieve equilibrium with its surroundings, it is subjected two opposite forces: a thermodynamic force of mixing of the hydrogel and the retractive force by the polymer chains. In other words, swelling is a function of the thermodynamic balance between polymer and water molecules and the elastic forces of the polymer chains. These forces are equal and opposite in equilibrium. An equilibrium situation of a neutral hydrogel can be stated regarding Gibbs free energy as:

$$\Delta G_{total} = \Delta G_{elastic} + \Delta G_{mixing} \tag{5.1}$$

Where, $\Delta G_{elastic}$ indicates the contribution from the elastic retractive forces established inside the network and ΔG_{mixing} is the measure of the compatibility between polymer and water molecules.

Mesh size of pores, i.e., the space between macromolecular chains, is another important structural parameter for analyzing hydrogel. Hydrogels can also be classifieds depending on the size of the pores as macroporous, microporous, or non-porous. The mesh size or correlation length (ζ) can be calculated using the following equation:

$$\zeta = a\overline{(r_0}^2)^{(1/2)} \tag{5.2}$$

Where, a is the elongation ratio of the polymer chain and $\overline{(r_0}^2)^{(1/2)}$ is the root mean square end-to-end distance between two consecutive cross-linking.

5.4 CHEMICAL SENSING BY STIMULI-RESPONSIVE HYDROGELS

5.4.1 TEMPERATURE SENSING

Temperature-sensitive (thermo-sensitive) polymers are extensively used as photonic crystal gels, as bulk hydrogels, in patterns, and in other different forms [49, 50].

Thermo-sensitive hydrogels utilizing temperature-sensitive polymers can be used as hydrogel photonic crystals (PCs), bulk hydrogel forms, and intelligent polymerized crystalline colloidal arrays (IPCCAs) for temperature sensing.

In PCs, dielectric constant varies, periodically creating a photonic band structure for electromagnetic waves to pass [51]. In any sensing application using PC, usually a variation in the periodic structure is probed. When a temperature-sensitive material is incorporated into a PC, it can be used for the detection of temperature. Kang et al. developed hydrogel based on hydroxyethyl methacrylate (HEMA) PCs for temperature sensors [52]. They constructed (using lithography and photoresist of hydrogel) three-dimensional hydrogel PCs where a change in temperature causes morphological changes in PCs as shown in Figure 5.2.

These changes were observed through the inversion caused by hydrogel PCs into silica structure. The changes in the lattice distance of the (111) direction during the swelling result in a shift of the photonic band concerning temperature.

IPCCA is made of a crystal colloidal array of polymer spheres that are polymerized in a hydrogel system [53]. The colloidal spheres diffract light, resulting in rising intense color. After combination with temperature-sensitive

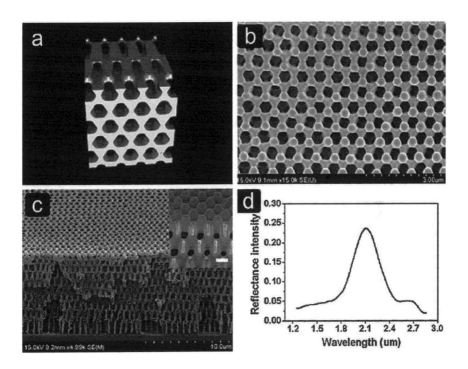

FIGURE 5.2 3D hydrogels: (a) interferential 3D holographic. (111) plane is at the front side. (b) Its SEM image and (c) 408 tilted cross-section in SEM image. Inset is the windows between lattices on the the (−1 1 0) plane. (d) The reflectance intensity of a nitrogen-dried hydrogel structure.

Source: Copyright permission from [52].

polymer, IPCCA turns into a suitable candidate for temperature sensing. An increase in temperature gives rise to an increase in the volume of the hydrogel, and the distance between two adjacent colloidal spheres changes. This increase in distance shifts the Bragg peak of reflected light to a longer wavelength [54].

Sun et al. have developed luminescent and fluorescent-based temperature probes which showed temperature-sensitive emission [55]. These probes are highly sensitive, inert to strong electric fields, and capable of operating contactless. Europium(III), a luminescent probe, has been incorporated into a hydrogel matrix for the detection of temperature [56].

5.4.2 IONS, IONIC STRENGTH, AND pH SENSING

In reaction to change in pH, pH-sensitive hydrogels reversibly show variation in their volume, mass, and elasticity and have promising applications in microsensors and microactuators in micro-electro-mechanical systems (MEMS) [57, 58]. The mechanisms for swelling dependent pH detection are the following: resonance frequency shift of a quartz crystal microbalance in microgravimetric sensors [59], change in the holographic diffraction wavelength in Bragg grating sensors [59], and the deflection of silicon membranes in piezoresistive pressure sensors [60].

Gerlach et al. utilized the swelling property of pH-responsive hydrogels by combining the piezoresistive-responsive elements with transition behavior of poly(vinyl alcohol)/poly(acrylic acid) (PVA/PAA) hydrogel [60]. A rapid responding photonic crystal pH sensor was developed by Shin et al. utilizing opal hydrogel structures [61]. Reese et al. constructed a hydrogel based on an IPCCA which swells/deswells when pH is changed due to protonation/deprotonation [62]. Kim and Beeb constructed pH-sensitive sensors on the basis of elastic volatilities of bi-polymer swelling hydrogels [63]. Maruyama et al. developed a method based on hydrogel to measure the local distribution of pH by a change in color [64].

Ion sensing by hydrogels applies the same principle as that of pH sensing. Guenther et al. fabricated an online analytical system for metal ion sensing by improving a rheochemical sensor on a piezoresistive pressure sensor chip which consisted of chemical and viscosity sensors [65]. Asher et al. modified IPCCA for Lead (Pb^{2+}) ion sensing [66]. A DNA hydrogel system was also used for Hg(II) detection [67]. Recently for the detection of both ionic strength and pH, hydrogel arrays consisting of perforated piezoresistive diaphragms were applied [68]. They were composed of three components: (i) piezoresistive sensor for ion detection, (ii) pH-sensitive hydrogel, and (iii) backing plate as shown in Figure 5.3. The backing plate was perforated, and the flow to hydrogel was made possible through diffusion pores. Change in pressure onto a piezoresistive sensor was induced by swelling/deswelling of hydrogels due to change in ion strength. This pressure change was converted directly into electrical signals.

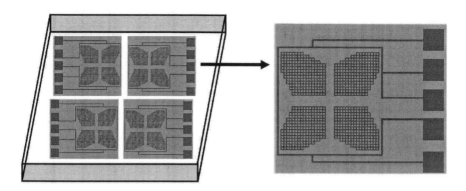

FIGURE 5.3 Schematic illustration of the perforated diaphragm pressure sensor array. Enlarged portion shows one of the 1 mm × 1 mm sensor designs.

Source: Based on [68].

5.4.3 Gas and Humidity Sensing

Hydrogel can be used for three purposes when applied in gas sensing for three reasons: first, its protein repellent and antiadhesive nature can be utilized by applying it as a passive protection coating for electrodes/sensors [69]; second, gas-sensitive molecules can be used to modify hydrogel (e.g., special fluorescent dye) to impart sensitiveness for certain gases [70]; third, its swelling characteristics can be used for gas sensing (e.g., carbon dioxide) using the Severinghaus principle [71].

Oh et al. developed a nitric oxide (NO) sensor by using hydrogel as a protective layer for planner ultramicroelectrode [72]. The gas-permeable membrane and the working electrode were distracted by an internal hydrogel layer. Zguris and Pishko fabricated a NO sensor which utilized 4-amino-5-methylamino-2',7'-difluorofluorescein (DAF-FM) entrapped within ploy(ethylene glycol) (PEG) hydrogel [73]. The swelling property of hydrogel was utilized for gas sensing by Herber et al. [74]. They fabricated a prototype of a continuous carbon dioxide (CO_2) sensor as development over standard air tonometry as represented in Figure 5.4. A pH-responsive hydrogel disk was secured between a pressure-sensitive membrane and a porous metal screen along with bicarbonate solution. pH changes with CO_2 reacted with the bicarbonate solution, which resulted in changing the pressure (a measure of the partial pressure of CO_2).

Humidity sensing is also significant in various industries such as petroleum, textiles, food, ceramics, etc. [75]. Mostly color change is observed in optical-based detection for humidity sensing [76] using a photonic crystal. Tian et al. developed a humidity sensitive hydrogel by incorporating the acrylamide (AAm) solution into a PC template [77]. Barry and Wiltzius fabricated a humidity sensor via polyacrylamide-based inverse opal hydrogel (IOH) that shifted its optical reflection peak significantly in response to humidity [78].

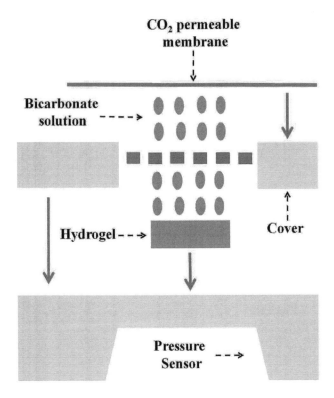

FIGURE 5.4   Schematic representation for PCO_2 sensor based on hydrogels.

Source: Modified from [74].

5.5   BIOCHEMICAL SENSING BY BIORESPONSIVE HYDROGELS

This section provides some examples of bioresponsive hydrogels in which biochemical properties of hydrogels have been improved by incorporating biological molecules (enzyme, antibody, nucleotide, oligonucleotide, etc.); these hydrogels have been used to detect different analytes (e.g., alcohol, amino acid, ammonia, glucose, hydrogen peroxide).

5.5.1   MOLECULAR INTERACTION

Biochemical sensing using hydrogel is achieved through different interaction mechanisms between the hydrogels and the analytes of interest, such as enzyme-analyte interaction, antibody-antigen interaction, etc.

5.5.1.1   Enzyme-Based Sensing

Alcohol: Wu et al. constructed an alcohol biosensor using hydrogel [79]. They co-incorporated alcohol oxidase and horseradish peroxidase (HRP) inside a polymer hydrogel matrix. Jang and Koh developed an alcohol sensor based on poly(ethylene glycol) (PEG) hydrogel in which multiplexed enzyme was employed within a micro-fluidic device [80]. They fabricated a model device for multiple sensing of alcohol and glucose by entrapping alcohol oxidase and glucose oxidase inside differently shaped hydrogel microparticles as shown in Figure 5.5. They serially connected the detection chamber (microfilter integrated) and two patterning chambers through a Y-shaped microchannel. The photolithography technique was used to fabricate the differently shaped hydrogel microplates, and pressure-driven flow was used to collect them in a detection chamber. Detection of glucose and alcohol simultaneously was performed through fluorescence imaging.

Amino acids: Hydrogel has also been used for the detection of amino acids. Castillo et al. fabricated a L-glutamate sensor by developing a bi-enzyme redox poly(1-vinylimidazole) (PVI) together with Os(4,4'-diethylbpy)$_2$Cl(termed PVI$_{19}$-demOs)/Poly(ethylene glycol)(400)diglycide ether (PEGDGE) hydrogel [81].

Ammonia: Kwan et al. constructed an ammonia sensor using poly(carbamoyl) sulfonate hydrogel matrix by co-incorporating glutamate oxidase and glutamate dehydrogenase on an oxygen electrode [82].

Glucose: Demand for glucose sensors has been rapidly enhanced in the last decades due to the rapid increase in the number of diabetes patients. Accordingly, the demand for hydrogel-based glucose sensors has also grown. Here we only focus on recent studies.

The most conventional method of glucose sensing is done by using glucose oxidase (GOX), or glucose dehydrogenase. Cai et al. exploited the swelling property of hydrogel by a mass-sensitive magnetoelastic sensor [83]. Mugweru et al. fabricated a glucose sensor by entrapping GOX into a poly(ethylene glycol) diacrylate (PEG-DA) hydrogel matrix [84]. Merchant et al. developed a highly sensitive

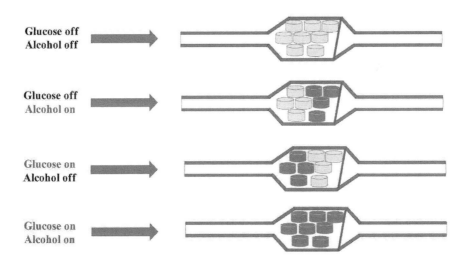

FIGURE 5.5 Recognition of ethanol and glucose using shape-coded hydrogel microparticles.
Source: Adapted from [80].

amperometric biosensor for glucose and hydrogen peroxide using cross-linked films of ferrocene-modified linear poly(ethylene amine) with immobilized GOX and horseradish peroxidase [85]. Glucose sensing was also made possible through optical sensing by Kim et al. [86]. They developed a self-assembled peptide hydrogel network containing nanofibers in which enzyme receptors (e.g., GOX or HRP) were physically encapsulated in combination with quantum dots (e.g., CdTe, CdSe). The first capable step taken towards glucose sensing through the electrochemical method was done by Siegrist et al. for in vivo operation [87]. They reported the exploitation of a unique polypeptide-based fluorescent glucose-sensitive system while equally providing remarkable accuracy at hypoglycemic levels. Glucose-sensitive, fluorescently labeled polypeptides were derivative of glucose binding proteins (GBPs) and were genetically improved by cysteine. This assisted the conjugation reaction for environmentally sensitive thiol-reactive fluorophore (N-[2-(1-maleimidyl) ethyl]-7-(diethylamino)coumarin-3-carboxamide (MDCC)). Fluorescent-labeled glucose binding proteins were casted in a hydrogel (polyacrylamide) matrix and positioned at the tip of an optical fiber to detect glucose continuously as represented in Figure 5.6.

Hydrogen peroxide: It is also clinically significant and has various industrial applications as an oxidizing, sterilizing, and bleaching agent. Detection of hydrogen peroxide takes significant priority in biological, environmental, and clinical studies and industries [88]. Kim et al. reported the detection of H_2O_2 using poly(ethylene glycol) hydrogel containing HRP based on an intracellular optical nanosensor [89]. Varma and Mattisson fabricated an amperometric H_2O_2 sensor in water and organic solvents [90]. They constructed a two-electrode system with hydrogel (30% polyacrylamide gel entrapping catalase) in a Teflon rod and platinum (Pt) electrode. Yan et al. were successful in detecting H_2O_2 through enzyme-based optical biosensors [91]. They constructed a microstructure, which acted as a sensing agent, using photolithographic patterning of a PEG hydrogel in which HRP was already incorporated. Amplex Red, oxidized to resorufin (fluorescent) as HRP reacted to H_2O_2, was immobilized within the PEG hydrogel along with enzymes. When H_2O_2 produced after mitogenic stimulation of macrophages, fluorescence appeared in the hydrogel microstructures as shown in Figure 5.7.

5.5.1.2 Antibody-Antigen

Antibody-antigen-based sensing is generally utilized in affinity-based sensors which are coupled with immunochemical reactions [92]. The basic working principle relies on the specific recognition of antigens (or antibodies) immobilized onto the transducer, which then produces signal depending on the concentration of the analyte. Antibody-antigen interaction-based sensors have drawn attention due to their high accuracy and low detection limit [93].

Carrigan et al. applied a quartz crystal microgravimetry with dissipation (QCM-D) technique for detection of cytokines [94]. They used polyethyleneimine (PEI) and carboxymethylcellulose (CMC) as a hydrogel. In this technique, the antibody was immobilized covalently via cross-linking between succinimide esters produced on the antibody and the carboxymethyl group of CMC. The hydrogel interface was utilized for the detection of cytokines rhIL-6, rhIL-1ra, and riIL-18BPa antigens. Guidi et al. performed the detection of a carcinogen insulin-like growth factor-1 (IGF-1) using the surface plasmon resonance

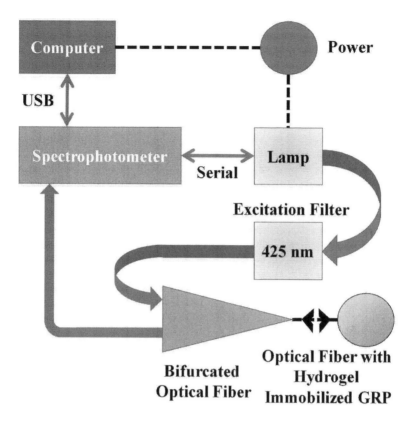

FIGURE 5.6 Detection of glucose by a hydrogel in the fiber-optic hardware system.
Source: Based on [87].

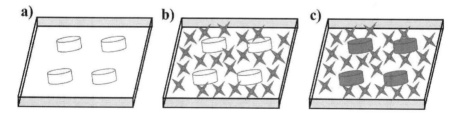

FIGURE 5.7 (a) PEG hydrogel micropatterns containing HRP, (b) seeding and culture of macrophages, and (c) release of H_2O_2 by macrophages by mitogenic stimulation.
Source: Based on [91].

(SPR) method [95]. Liang et al. applied the electrochemical-based sensing technique using three-dimensional porous chitosan hydrogel for hepatitis B surface antigen [96]. A designer nanocomposite solution of chitosan containing silica nanoparticles was electrodeposited on an ITO electrode. A porous network was prepared by the removal of silica nanoparticles. Hepatitis B surface antibody

(HBsAb) was covalently immobilized onto the hydrogel to detect Hepatitis B surface antigen.

5.5.1.3 Nucleotide, Oligonucleotide, and DNA

Nucleic acid detection has become very significant due to the importance of forensic analysis and genetic and disease diagnosis [97]. Electrochemical, fluorescence, optical, microgravtometric, and electrical systems have been extensively used for the detection of DNA [98–100]. Due to advanced immobilization ability to sense moieties, hydrogel-based systems result in hundredfold signal density [101]. Due to their hydrophilic nature, flexible structure, and high water-swollen capacity hydrogels do not tend to perturb the thermodynamically stable form of nucleic.

Microcantilever is one of the widely applied tools for DNA sensing. Hydrogel-coated cantilevers hold together the properties of hydrogel and immobilized probes as well as avoids non-specific binding interaction of probe to achieve high accuracy and sensitivity. Keov et al. developed a cantilever by electrodepositing chitosan for nucleic acid hybridization detection [102]. In the field of DNA detection, very often DNA microarrays are used. Seong et al. constructed DNA hybridization using microchannels in combination with photolithography-defined wires and UV-cross-linked hydrogel [103]. An array platform consisting of specific analyte indexed by shape was fabricated with poly(ethylene glycol) acrylate hydrogel by Meiring et al. [104].

5.5.2 LIVING SENSORS

The utilization of hydrogel in combination with living cells and microorganisms for biosensing has also been researched in the last decade. Living cells have been immobilized in different types of hydrogels such as chitosan, poly(ethylene glycol), polyvinyl alcohol, polyacrylamide, alginate, photo cross-linkable resins, low-melting agarose, proteinic matrix, and polyacrylonitrile membranes [105–115]. The three-dimensional network and large water content of the hydrogels facilitate in transporting nutrition into cells and high gas exchange rate. Biocompatibility along with the aforementioned properties of hydrogels even allow cultivating bacteria or cells inside the hydrogel, which can be further utilized as a platform for biosensing applications.

5.5.2.1 Bacteria

Renneberg et al. used bacteria as biological recognition elements for the rapid detection of pollutants in the wastewater body [116]. They took poly(carbamoyl)sulfonate (PCS) hydrogel on a Clark-type electrode in which yeast *Arxulaadeninivorans* LS3 cells were immobilized as represented in Figure 5.8. Fine et al. constructed fiber-optic biosensors using calcium alginate or polyvinylalcohol (PVA) entrapping luminescent yeast cells for the biodetection of estrogenic endocrine-disrupting chemical (EDC) [117]. The protective hydrogel matrix made it possible to even detect under non-sterile environments. Koster et al. used polyurethane hydrogel to immobilize aerobic seawater microorganisms (related to *Staphylococcus warneri*) for the detection of available dissolved organic carbon (ADOC) [118]. Fesenko et al. constructed

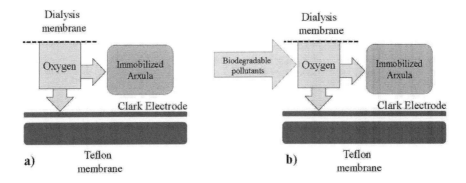

FIGURE 5.8 Schematic of the *A. adeninivorans* LS3 microbial sensor: (a) microbial consumption of oxygen before and (b) addition of biodegradable pollutants.

Source: Modified from [116].

a polyacrylamide hydrogel-based bacterial microchip (HBMChip) using *E. coli* for the detection and monitoring of cell pollutants [119].

5.5.2.2 Cells

Hydrogels offer in vitro and in vivo applications due to having a structural resemblance to the cellular microenvironment (extracellular matrix) in the human body. Hydrogels are used either as a 3D matrix for cells or coating material for biological recognition elements. Ding et al. developed a nanocomposite gel using chitosan-encapsulated gold nanoparticles for electrochemical study and immobilization of cells (K562 leukemia cells), which monitors their proliferation, adhesion, and apoptosis on electrode [120]. Kim et al. fabricated patterned poly(ethylene glycol) dimethacrylate (PEGDMA) hydrogels microwells using T-cells and B-cells for the detection of the pathogen in chip format [17]. Using a collagen matrix, Banerjee et al. constructed a multiwell plate-based sensor encapsulating B-cell, Ped-2E9 for pathogenic detection (*Listeria*) [121].

5.6 CONCLUSION AND FUTURE PERSPECTIVE

Hydrogels have found themselves widely applicable in the field of sensing due to their intrinsic characteristics, such as high water content, biocompatibility, and easy functionalization with different recognition elements. Stimuli-sensitive and bioresponsive hydrogels are specially designed from natural and synthetic hydrogels for specific detection of analytes and species. The future success in sensing applications using hydrogels depends on the novelty of these designed hydrogels which can address the medical challenges. Future developments in hydrogels will come through precise macromolecular chemistry to tune size, structure, shape, and basic building blocks of hydrogels. With modern biotechnological tools, the synthesis and design of stimuli-sensitive and bioresponsive hydrogels with uncompromised sensitivity and accuracy will be very promising.

REFERENCES

[1] E.M. Ahmed, Hydrogel: Preparation, characterization, and applications: A review, *Journal of Advanced Research*, 6 (2015) 105–121.

[2] B. Xing, C-W. Yu, K-H. Chow, P-L. Ho, D. Fu, B. Xu, Hydrophobic interaction and hydrogen bonding cooperatively confer a vancomycin hydrogel: A potential candidate for biomaterials, *Journal of the American Chemical Society*, 124 (2002) 14846–14847.

[3] Z. Yang, H. Gu, D. Fu, P. Gao, J.K. Lam, B. Xu, Enzymatic formation of supramolecular hydrogels, *Advanced Materials*, 16 (2004) 1440–1444.

[4] B.D. Ratner, A.S. Hoffman, F.J. Schoen, J.E. Lemons, *Biomaterials Science: An Introduction to Materials in Medicine*, Elsevier, 2004.

[5] K. Abdel-Halim, A. Salama, E. El-Khateeb, N. Bakry, Organophosphorus pollutants (OPP) in aquatic environment at Damietta Governorate, Egypt: Implications for monitoring and biomarker responses, *Chemosphere*, 63 (2006) 1491–1498.

[6] F.L. Buchholz, A.T. Graham, *Modern Superabsorbent Polymer Technology*, John! Wiley & Sons, Inc, 605 Third Ave, New York, NY 10016, 1998, 279.

[7] Y. Li, G. Huang, X. Zhang, B. Li, Y. Chen, T. Lu, T.J. Lu, F. Xu, Magnetic hydrogels and their potential biomedical applications, *Advanced Functional Materials*, 23 (2013) 660–672.

[8] J. Groll, E.V. Amirgoulova, T. Ameringer, C.D. Heyes, C. Röcker, G.U. Nienhaus, M. Möller, Biofunctionalized, ultrathin coatings of cross-linked star-shaped poly (ethylene oxide) allow reversible folding of immobilized proteins, *Journal of the American Chemical Society*, 126 (2004) 4234–4239.

[9] P. Gasteier, A. Reska, P. Schulte, J. Salber, A. Offenhäusser, M. Moeller, J. Groll, Surface grafting of PEO-based star-shaped molecules for bioanalytical and biomedical applications, *Macromolecular Bioscience*, 7 (2007) 1010–1023.

[10] V. Alzari, O. Monticelli, D. Nuvoli, J.M. Kenny, A. Mariani, Stimuli responsive hydrogels prepared by frontal polymerization, *Biomacromolecules*, 10 (2009) 2672–2677.

[11] M. Casolaro, E. Paccagnini, R. Mendichi, Y. Ito, Stimuli-responsive polymers based on L-phenylalanine residues: Protonation thermodynamics of free polymers and cross-linked hydrogels, *Macromolecules*, 38 (2005) 2460–2468.

[12] S. Garty, N. Kimelman-Bleich, Z. Hayouka, D. Cohn, A. Friedler, G. Pelled, D. Gazit, Peptide-modified "smart" hydrogels and genetically engineered stem cells for skeletal tissue engineering, *Biomacromolecules*, 11 (2010) 1516–1526.

[13] H. Wei, H. Yu, A-Y. Zhang, L-G. Sun, D. Hou, Z-G. Feng, Synthesis and characterization of thermosensitive and supramolecular structured hydrogels, *Macromolecules*, 38 (2005) 8833–8839.

[14] V.L. Alexeev, A.C. Sharma, A.V. Goponenko, S. Das, I.K. Lednev, C.S. Wilcox, D.N. Finegold, S.A. Asher, High ionic strength glucose-sensing photonic crystal, *Analytical Chemistry*, 75 (2003) 2316–2323.

[15] J. Kim, S. Nayak, L.A. Lyon, Bioresponsive hydrogel microlenses, *Journal of the American Chemical Society*, 127 (2005) 9588–9592.

[16] Z. Yang, P-L. Ho, G. Liang, K.H. Chow, Q. Wang, Y. Cao, Z. Guo, B. Xu, Using β-lactamase to trigger supramolecular hydrogelation, *Journal of the American Chemical Society*, 129 (2007) 266–267.

[17] H. Kim, R.E. Cohen, P.T. Hammond, D.J. Irvine, Live lymphocyte arrays for biosensing, *Advanced Functional Materials*, 16 (2006) 1313–1323.

[18] F. Topuz, O. Okay, Formation of hydrogels by simultaneous denaturation and cross-linking of DNA, *Biomacromolecules*, 10 (2009) 2652–2661.

[19] K. Trabbic-Carlson, L.A. Setton, A. Chilkoti, Swelling and mechanical behaviors of chemically cross-linked hydrogels of elastin-like polypeptides, *Biomacromolecules*, 4 (2003) 572–580.

[20] N. Sanabria-DeLong, A.J. Crosby, G.N. Tew, Photo-cross-linked PLA-PEO-PLA hydrogels from self-assembled physical networks: Mechanical properties and influence of assumed constitutive relationships, *Biomacromolecules*, 9 (2008) 2784–2791.

[21] M.C. Branco, F. Nettesheim, D.J. Pochan, J.P. Schneider, N.J. Wagner, Fast dynamics of semiflexible chain networks of self-assembled peptides, *Biomacromolecules*, 10 (2009) 1374–1380.

[22] Z. Maolin, L. Jun, Y. Min, H. Hongfei, The swelling behavior of radiation prepared semi-interpenetrating polymer networks composed of polyNIPAAm and hydrophilic polymers, *Radiation Physics and Chemistry*, 58 (2000) 397–400.

[23] E. Merrill, E. Salzman, S. Wan, N. Mahmud, L. Kushner, J. Lindon, J. Curme, Platelet-compatible hydrophilic segmented polyurethanes from polyethylene glycols and cyclohexane diisocyanate, *Transactions-American Society for Artificial Internal Organs*, 28 (1982) 482–487.

[24] G.M. Whitesides, E. Ostuni, S. Takayama, X. Jiang, D.E. Ingber, Soft lithography in biology and biochemistry, *Annual Review of Biomedical Engineering*, 3 (2001) 335–373.

[25] S. Lu, K.S. Anseth, Photopolymerization of multilaminated poly (HEMA) hydrogels for controlled release, *Journal of Controlled Release*, 57 (1999) 291–300.

[26] A. Kidane, J.M. Szabocsik, K. Park, Accelerated study on lysozyme deposition on poly (HEMA) contact lenses, *Biomaterials*, 19 (1998) 2051–2055.

[27] N.A. Peppas, E.W. Merrill, Development of semicrystalline poly (vinyl alcohol) hydrogels for biomedical applications, *Journal of Biomedical Materials Research*, 11 (1977) 423–434.

[28] P.J. Martens, S.J. Bryant, K.S. Anseth, Tailoring the degradation of hydrogels formed from multivinyl poly (ethylene glycol) and poly (vinyl alcohol) macromers for cartilage tissue engineering, *Biomacromolecules*, 4 (2003) 283–292.

[29] S.M. Shaheen, K. Yamaura, Preparation of theophylline hydrogels of atactic poly (vinyl alcohol)/NaCl/H2O system for drug delivery system, *Journal of Controlled Release*, 81 (2002) 367–377.

[30] N.A. Peppas, A.R. Khare, Preparation, structure and diffusional behavior of hydrogels in controlled release, *Advanced Drug Delivery Reviews*, 11 (1993) 1–35.

[31] A.R. Khare, N.A. Peppas, Release behavior of bioactive agents from pH-sensitive hydrogels, *Journal of Biomaterials Science, Polymer Edition*, 4 (1993) 275–289.

[32] R.A. Scott, N.A. Peppas, Kinetics of copolymerization of PEG-containing multiacrylates with acrylic acid, *Macromolecules*, 32 (1999) 6149–6158.

[33] B. Jeong, S.W. Kim, Y.H. Bae, Thermosensitive sol—gel reversible hydrogels, *Advanced Drug Delivery Reviews*, 64 (2012) 154–162.

[34] S. Sershen, J. West, corrigendum to: "Implantable, polymeric systems for modulated drug delivery." [*Advanced Drug Delivery Reviews*, 54 (2002) 1225–1235]☆, *Advanced Drug Delivery Reviews*, 55 (2003) 439.

[35] E.S. Gil, S.M. Hudson, Stimuli-reponsive polymers and their bioconjugates, *Progress in Polymer Science*, 29 (2004) 1173–1222.

[36] K. Podual, F.J. Doyle III, N.A. Peppas, Glucose-sensitivity of glucose oxidase-containing cationic copolymer hydrogels having poly (ethylene glycol) grafts, *Journal of Controlled Release*, 67 (2000) 9–17.

[37] J.D. Ehrick, S.K. Deo, T.W. Browning, L.G. Bachas, M.J. Madou, S. Daunert, Genetically engineered protein in hydrogels tailors stimuli-responsive characteristics, *Nature Materials*, 4 (2005) 298.

[38] J.A. Burdick, A. Khademhosseini, R. Langer, Fabrication of gradient hydrogels using a microfluidics/photopolymerization process, *Langmuir*, 20 (2004) 5153–5156.

[39] K.S. Anseth, A.T. Metters, S.J. Bryant, P.J. Martens, J.H. Elisseeff, C.N. Bowman, In situ forming degradable networks and their application in tissue engineering and drug delivery, *Journal of Controlled Release*, 78 (2002) 199–209.

[40] B.K. Mann, R.H. Schmedlen, J.L. West, Tethered-TGF-β increases extracellular matrix production of vascular smooth muscle cells, *Biomaterials*, 22 (2001) 439–444.

[41] S. Zhang, Fabrication of novel biomaterials through molecular self-assembly, *Nature Biotechnology*, 21 (2003) 1171.

[42] B. Sellergren, Noncovalent molecular imprinting: Antibody-like molecular recognition in polymeric network materials, *TrAC Trends in Analytical Chemistry*, 16 (1997) 310–320.

[43] M.E. Byrne, E. Oral, J. Zachary Hilt, N.A. Peppas, Networks for recognition of biomolecules: Molecular imprinting and micropatterning poly (ethylene glycol)-Containing films, *Polymers for Advanced Technologies*, 13 (2002) 798–816.

[44] M.E. Byrne, K. Park, N.A. Peppas, Molecular imprinting within hydrogels, *Advanced Drug Delivery Reviews*, 54 (2002) 149–161.

[45] S. Eichler, O. Ramon, Y. Cohen, S. Mizrahi, Swelling and contraction driven mass transfer processes during osmotic dehydration of uncharged hydrogels, *International Journal of Food Science & Technology*, 37 (2002) 245–253.

[46] F. Ganji, F.S. Vasheghani, F.E. Vasheghani, Theoretical description of hydrogel swelling: A review (2010).

[47] R.A. Gemeinhart, C. Guo, 13 Fast swelling hydrogel systems, reflexive polymers and hydrogels: Understanding and designing fast responsive polymeric systems (2004) 245.

[48] R. Langer, N.A. Peppas, Advances in biomaterials, drug delivery, and bionanotechnology, *AIChE Journal*, 49 (2003) 2990–3006.

[49] D. Kuckling, Responsive hydrogel layers—from synthesis to applications, *Colloid and Polymer Science*, 287 (2009) 881–891.

[50] M.A.C. Stuart, W.T. Huck, J. Genzer, M. Müller, C. Ober, M. Stamm, G.B. Sukhorukov, I. Szleifer, V.V. Tsukruk, M. Urban, Emerging applications of stimuli-responsive polymer materials, *Nature Materials*, 9 (2010) 101.

[51] R.V. Nair, R. Vijaya, Photonic crystal sensors: An overview, *Progress in Quantum Electronics*, 34 (2010) 89–134.

[52] J.H. Kang, J.H. Moon, S.K. Lee, S.G. Park, S.G. Jang, S. Yang, S.M. Yang, Thermoresponsive hydrogel photonic crystals by three-dimensional holographic lithography, *Advanced Materials*, 20 (2008) 3061–3065.

[53] J.P. Walker, K.W. Kimble, S.A. Asher, Photonic crystal sensor for organophosphate nerve agents utilizing the organophosphorus hydrolase enzyme, *Analytical and Bioanalytical Chemistry*, 389 (2007) 2115–2124.

[54] S.A. Asher, J. Holtz, L. Liu, Z. Wu, Self-assembly motif for creating submicron periodic materials: Polymerized crystalline colloidal arrays, *Journal of the American Chemical Society*, 116 (1994) 4997–4998.

[55] L-N. Sun, J. Yu, H. Peng, J.Z. Zhang, L-Y. Shi, O.S. Wolfbeis, Temperature-sensitive luminescent nanoparticles and films based on a terbium (III) complex probe, *The Journal of Physical Chemistry C*, 114 (2010) 12642–12648.

[56] P. Schrenkhammer, I.C. Rosnizeck, A. Duerkop, O.S. Wolfbeis, M. Schäferling, Time-resolved fluorescence-based assay for the determination of alkaline phosphatase activity and application to the screening of its inhibitors, *Journal of Biomolecular Screening*, 13 (2008) 9–16.

[57] D. Kuckling, A. Richter, K.F. Arndt, Temperature and pH-dependent swelling behavior of poly (N-isopropylacrylamide) copolymer hydrogels and their use in flow control, *Macromolecular Materials and Engineering*, 288 (2003) 144–151.

[58] K.F. Arndt, A. Richter, S. Ludwig, J. Zimmermann, J. Kressler, D. Kuckling, H.J. Adler, Poly (vinyl alcohol)/poly (acrylic acid) hydrogels: FT-IR spectroscopic characterization of crosslinking reaction and work at transition point, *Acta Polymerica*, 50 (1999) 383–390.

[59] A. Richter, A. Bund, M. Keller, K-F. Arndt, Characterization of a microgravimetric sensor based on pH sensitive hydrogels, *Sensors and Actuators B: Chemical*, 99 (2004) 579–585.

[60] G. Gerlach, M. Guenther, G. Suchaneck, J. Sorber, K.F. Arndt, A. Richter, Application of sensitive hydrogels in chemical and pH sensors, in: *Macromolecular Symposia, Wiley Online Library*, 2004, pp. 403–410.

[61] J. Shin, P.V. Braun, W. Lee, Fast response photonic crystal pH sensor based on templated photo-polymerized hydrogel inverse opal, *Sensors and Actuators B: Chemical*, 150 (2010) 183–190.

[62] C.E. Reese, M.E. Baltusavich, J.P. Keim, S.A. Asher, Development of an intelligent polymerized crystalline colloidal array colorimetric reagent, *Analytical Chemistry*, 73 (2001) 5038–5042.

[63] D. Kim, D.J. Beebe, A sensing method based on elastic instabilities of swelllng hydrogels, in: *International Conference on Microtechnologies in Medicine and Biology*, IEEE, 2006, pp. 292–294.

[64] H. Maruyama, H. Matsumoto, T. Fukuda, F. Arai, Functionalized hydrogel surface patterned in a chip for local pH sensing, in: *IEEE 21st International Conference on Micro Electro Mechanical Systems*, MEMS, IEEE, 2008, pp. 224–227.

[65] M. Guenther, G. Gerlach, C. Corten, D. Kuckling, J. Sorber, K-F. Arndt, Hydrogel-based sensor for a rheochemical characterization of solutions, *Sensors and Actuators B: Chemical*, 132 (2008) 471–476.

[66] S.A. Asher, S.F. Peteu, C.E. Reese, M. Lin, D. Finegold, Polymerized crystalline colloidal array chemical-sensing materials for detection of lead in body fluids, *Analytical and Bioanalytical Chemistry*, 373 (2002) 632–638.

[67] A. Baeissa, N. Dave, B.D. Smith, J. Liu, DNA-functionalized monolithic hydrogels and gold nanoparticles for colorimetric DNA detection, *ACS Applied Materials & Interfaces*, 2 (2010) 3594–3600.

[68] M. Orthner, G. Lin, M. Avula, S. Buetefisch, J. Magda, L. Rieth, F. Solzbacher, Hydrogel based sensor arrays (2× 2) with perforated piezoresistive diaphragms for metabolic monitoring (in vitro), *Sensors and Actuators B: Chemical*, 145 (2010) 807–816.

[69] J. Hart, A. Abass, A disposable amperometric gas sensor for Sulphur-containing compounds based on a chemically modified screen printed carbon electrode coated with a hydrogel, *Analytica Chimica Acta*, 342 (1997) 199–206.

[70] J. Kojima, Y. Nakayama, M. Takenaka, T. Hashimoto, Apparatus for measuring time-resolved light scattering profiles from supercritical polymer solutions undergoing phase separation under high pressure, *Review of Scientific Instruments*, 66 (1995) 4066–4072.

[71] J.W. Severinghaus, First electrodes for blood PO2 and PCO2 determination, *Journal of Applied Physiology*, 97 (2004) 1599–1600.

[72] B.K. Oh, M.E. Robbins, M.H. Schoenfisch, Planar nitric oxide (NO)-selective ultramicroelectrode sensor for measuring localized NO surface concentrations at xerogel microarrays, *Analyst*, 131 (2006) 48–54.

[73] J. Zguris, M.V. Pishko, Nitric oxide sensitive fluorescent poly (ethylene glycol) hydrogel microstructures, *Sensors and Actuators B: Chemical*, 115 (2006) 503–509.

[74] S. Herber, W. Olthuis, P. Bergveld, A. van den Berg, Exploitation of a pH-sensitive hydrogel disk for CO2 detection, *Sensors and Actuators B: Chemical*, 103 (2004) 284–289.

[75] J-W. Rhim, Increase in water vapor barrier property of biopolymer-based edible films and coatings by compositing with lipid materials, *Food Science and Biotechnology*, 13 (2004) 528–535.

[76] F. García-Golding, M. Giallorenzo, N. Moreno, V. Chang, Sensor for determining the water content of oil-in-water emulsion by specific admittance measurement, *Sensors and Actuators A: Physical*, 47 (1995) 337–341.

[77] E. Tian, J. Wang, Y. Zheng, Y. Song, L. Jiang, D. Zhu, Colorful humidity sensitive photonic crystal hydrogel, *Journal of Materials Chemistry*, 18 (2008) 1116–1122.

[78] R.A. Barry, P. Wiltzius, Humidity-sensing inverse opal hydrogels, *Langmuir*, 22 (2006) 1369–1374.

[79] X.J. Wu, M.M. Choi, C.S. Chen, X.M. Wu, On-line monitoring of methanol in n-hexane by an organic-phase alcohol biosensor, *Biosensors and Bioelectronics*, 22 (2007) 1337–1344.

[80] E. Jang, W-G. Koh, Multiplexed enzyme-based bioassay within microfluidic devices using shape-coded hydrogel microparticles, *Sensors and Actuators B: Chemical*, 143 (2010) 681–688.

[81] J. Castillo, A. Blöchl, S. Dennison, W. Schuhmann, E. Csöregi, Glutamate detection from nerve cells using a planar electrodes array integrated in a microtiter plate, *Biosensors and Bioelectronics*, 20 (2005) 2116–2119.

[82] R.C. Kwan, P.Y. Hon, R. Renneberg, Amperometric determination of ammonium with bienzyme/poly (carbamoyl) sulfonate hydrogel-based biosensor, *Sensors and Actuators B: Chemical*, 107 (2005) 616–622.

[83] Q. Cai, K. Zeng, C. Ruan, T.A. Desai, C.A. Grimes, A wireless, remote query glucose biosensor based on a pH-sensitive polymer, *Analytical Chemistry*, 76 (2004) 4038–4043.

[84] A. Mugweru, B.L. Clark, M.V. Pishko, Electrochemical sensor array for glucose monitoring fabricated by rapid immobilization of active glucose oxidase within photochemically polymerized hydrogels, *Journal of Diabetes Science and Technology*, 1 (2007) 366–371.

[85] S.A. Merchant, T.O. Tran, M.T. Meredith, T.C. Cline, D.T. Glatzhofer, D.W. Schmidtke, High-sensitivity amperometric biosensors based on ferrocene-modified linear poly (ethylenimine), *Langmuir*, 25 (2009) 7736–7742.

[86] J.H. Kim, S.Y. Lim, D.H. Nam, J. Ryu, S.H. Ku, C.B. Park, Self-assembled, photoluminescent peptide hydrogel as a versatile platform for enzyme-based optical biosensors, *Biosensors and Bioelectronics*, 26 (2011) 1860–1865.

[87] J. Siegrist, T. Kazarian, C. Ensor, S. Joel, M. Madou, P. Wang, S. Daunert, Continuous glucose sensor using novel genetically engineered binding polypeptides towards in vivo applications, *Sensors and Actuators B: Chemical*, 149 (2010) 51–58.

[88] M. Aizawa, I. Karube, S. Suzuki, A specific bio-electrochemical sensor for hydrogen peroxide, *Analytica Chimica Acta*, 69 (1974) 431–437.

[89] S-H. Kim, B. Kim, V.K. Yadavalli, M.V. Pishko, Encapsulation of enzymes within polymer spheres to create optical nanosensors for oxidative stress, *Analytical Chemistry*, 77 (2005) 6828–6833.

[90] S. Varma, B. Mattiasson, Amperometric biosensor for the detection of hydrogen peroxide using catalase modified electrodes in polyacrylamide, *Journal of Biotechnology*, 119 (2005) 172–180.

[91] J. Yan, Y. Sun, H. Zhu, L. Marcu, A. Revzin, Enzyme-containing hydrogel micropatterns serving a dual purpose of cell sequestration and metabolite detection, *Biosensors and Bioelectronics*, 24 (2009) 2604–2610.

[92] J.M. Fowler, D.K. Wong, H.B. Halsall, W.R. Heineman, Recent developments in electrochemical immunoassays and immunosensors (2008).

[93] S. Laschi, M. Fránek, M. Mascini, Screen-printed electrochemical immunosensors for PCB detection, *Electroanalysis: An International Journal Devoted to Fundamental and Practical Aspects of Electroanalysis*, 12 (2000) 1293–1298.

[94] S.D. Carrigan, G. Scott, M. Tabrizian, Rapid three-dimensional biointerfaces for real-time immunoassay using hIL-18BPa as a model antigen, *Biomaterials*, 26 (2005) 7514–7523.

[95] A. Guidi, L. Laricchia-Robbio, D. Gianfaldoni, R. Revoltella, G. Del Bono, Comparison of a conventional immunoassay (ELISA) with a surface plasmon resonance-based biosensor for IGF-1 detection in cows' milk, *Biosensors and Bioelectronics*, 16 (2001) 971–977.

[96] R. Liang, H. Peng, J. Qiu, Fabrication, characterization, and application of potentiometric immunosensor based on biocompatible and controllable three-dimensional porous chitosan membranes, *Journal of Colloid and Interface Science*, 320 (2008) 125–131.

[97] Z.S. Wu, J.H. Jiang, G.L. Shen, R.Q. Yu, Highly sensitive DNA detection and point mutation identification: An electrochemical approach based on the combined use of ligase and reverse molecular beacon, *Human Mutation*, 28 (2007) 630–637.

[98] J. Wang, Electrochemical biosensors: Towards point-of-care cancer diagnostics, *Biosensors and Bioelectronics*, 21 (2006) 1887–1892.

[99] K.J. Odenthal, J.J. Gooding, An introduction to electrochemical DNA biosensors, *Analyst*, 132 (2007) 603–610.

[100] J.M. Kinsella, A. Ivanisevic, Biosensing: Taking charge of biomolecules, *Nature Nanotechnology*, 2 (2007) 596.

[101] D. Guschin, G. Yershov, A. Zaslavsky, A. Gemmell, V. Shick, D. Proudnikov, P. Arenkov, A. Mirzabekov, Manual manufacturing of oligonucleotide, DNA, and protein microchips, *Analytical Biochemistry*, 250 (1997) 203–211.

[102] S.T. Koev, M.A. Powers, H. Yi, L-Q. Wu, W.E. Bentley, G.W. Rubloff, G.F. Payne, R. Ghodssi, Mechano-transduction of DNA hybridization and dopamine oxidation through electrodeposited chitosan network, *Lab on a Chip*, 7 (2007) 103–111.

[103] G.H. Seong, W. Zhan, R.M. Crooks, Fabrication of microchambers defined by photopolymerized hydrogels and weirs within microfluidic systems: Application to DNA hybridization, *Analytical Chemistry*, 74 (2002) 3372–3377.

[104] J.E. Meiring, M.J. Schmid, S.M. Grayson, B.M. Rathsack, D.M. Johnson, R. Kirby, R. Kannappan, K. Manthiram, B. Hsia, Z.L. Hogan, Hydrogel biosensor array platform indexed by shape, *Chemistry of Materials*, 16 (2004) 5574–5580.

[105] A. Deshpande, S. D'souza, G. Nadkarni, Coimmobilization of D-amino acid oxidase and catalase by entrapment ofTrigonopsis variabilis in radiation polymerised Polyacrylamide beads, *Journal of Biosciences*, 11 (1987) 137–144.

[106] J. Peter, W. Hutter, W. Stöllnberger, W. Hampel, Detection of chlorinated and brominated hydrocarbons by an ion sensitive whole cell biosensor, *Biosensors and Bioelectronics*, 11 (1996) 1215–1219.

[107] A. König, C. Zaborosch, F. Spener, Microbial sensor for Pah in aqueous solution using solubilizers, in: *Field Screening Europe*, Springer, New York, 1997, pp. 203–206.

[108] S. Fukui, K. Sonomoto, A. Tanaka, [20] Entrapment of biocatalysts with photo-cross-linkable resin prepolymers and urethane resin prepolymers, in: *Methods in Enzymology*, Elsevier, 1987, pp. 230–252.

[109] Z. Yang, S. Sasaki, I. Karube, H. Suzuki, Fabrication of oxygen electrode arrays and their incorporation into sensors for measuring biochemical oxygen demand, *Analytica Chimica Acta*, 357 (1997) 41–49.

[110] R. Rouillon, M. Sole, R. Carpentier, J-L. Marty, Immobilization of thylakoids in polyvinylalcohol for the detection of herbicides, *Sensors and Actuators B: Chemical*, 27 (1995) 477–479.

[111] T. Uhlich, M. Ulbricht, G. Tomaschewski, Immobilization of enzymes in photochemically cross-linked polyvinyl alcohol, *Enzyme and Microbial Technology*, 19 (1996) 124–131.

[112] K. Tag, M. Lehmann, C. Chan, R. Renneberg, K. Riedel, G. Kunze, Measurement of biodegradable substances with a mycelia-sensor based on the salt tolerant yeast Arxula adeninivorans LS3, *Sensors and Actuators B: Chemical*, 67 (2000) 142–148.

[113] M. Ulbricht, A. Papra, Polyacrylonitrile enzyme ultrafiltration membranes prepared by adsorption, cross-linking, and covalent binding, *Enzyme and Microbial Technology*, 20 (1997) 61–68.

[114] J. Peter, W. Hutter, W. Stöllnberger, F. Karner, W. Hampel, Semicontinuous detection of 1, 2-dichloroethane in water samples using Xanthobacter autotrophicus GJ 10 encapsulated in chitosan beads, *Analytical Chemistry*, 69 (1997) 2077–2079.

[115] S.F. D'Souza, K.Z. Marolia, Stabilization of Micrococcus lysodeikticus cells towards lysis by lysozyme using glutaraldehyde: Application as a novel biospecific ligand for the purification of lysozyme, *Biotechnology Techniques*, 13 (1999) 375–378.

[116] T. Renneberg, R.C. Kwan, C. Chan, G. Kunze, R. Renneberg, A salt-tolerant yeast-based microbial sensor for 24 hour community wastewater monitoring in coastal regions, *Microchimica Acta*, 148 (2004) 235–240.

[117] T. Fine, P. Leskinen, T. Isobe, H. Shiraishi, M. Morita, R. Marks, M. Virta, Luminescent yeast cells entrapped in hydrogels for estrogenic endocrine disrupting chemical biodetection, *Biosensors and Bioelectronics*, 21 (2006) 2263–2269.

[118] M. Köster, C.G. Gliesche, R. Wardenga, Microbiosensors for measurement of microbially available dissolved organic carbon: Sensor characteristics and preliminary environmental application, *Applied and Environmental Microbiology*, 72 (2006) 7063–7073.

[119] D. Fesenko, T. Nasedkina, D. Prokopenko, A. Mirzabekov, Biosensing and monitoring of cell populations using the hydrogel bacterial microchip, *Biosensors and Bioelectronics*, 20 (2005) 1860–1865.

[120] L. Ding, C. Hao, Y. Xue, H. Ju, A bio-inspired support of gold nanoparticles– chitosan nanocomposites gel for immobilization and electrochemical study of K562 Leukemia cells, *Biomacromolecules*, 8 (2007) 1341–1346.

[121] P. Banerjee, D. Lenz, J.P. Robinson, J.L. Rickus, A.K. Bhunia, A novel and simple cell-based detection system with a collagen-encapsulated B-lymphocyte cell line as a biosensor for rapid detection of pathogens and toxins, *Laboratory Investigation*, 88 (2008) 196.

6 Biomedical Application of Hydrogels and Their Importance

Abhijeet Mishra, Anujit Ghosal,
Rangnath Ravi, and Namita Singh

CONTENTS

6.1 INTRODUCTION

Hydrogels are made up of polymers that can expand and swell but don't dissolve aqueous solutions (up to a certain limit) [1]. It is observed as colloidal suspension with water along with a dispersal medium [1, 2]. It retains water because these are made up of monomers with hydrophilic functional groups. However, it does not dissolve in water because of cross-links between the network chains [2]. Further, these networks maintain stability with the surrounding media and temperature for shape and strength [1, 2]. Hydrogels may be natural or may be synthetically synthesized in

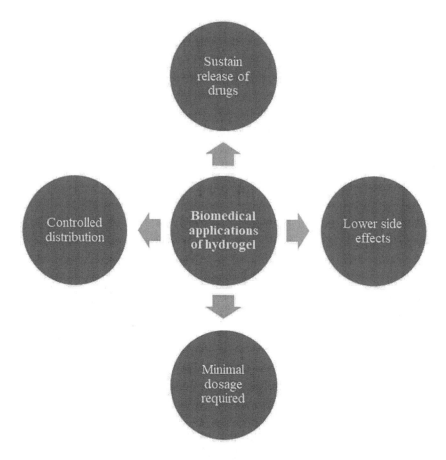

FIGURE 6.1 Importance of hydrogels in the biomedical arena.

the laboratories. The structure of hydrogels change if we alters the basic structure of monomers, cross-linker(s), and concentration. [3]. Hydrogels can be used in different fields including biomedical science (Figure 6.1).

6.2 PROPERTIES OF HYDROGELS

1) **Swelling:** Swelling is the most important characteristic of a hydrogel. These structures support free diffusion of solute molecules in aqueous media while the polymer network of hydrogel functions as a vessel to hold the solvent jointly together. They can absorb up to thousands of times their dry weight in liquid media [4].

2) **Permeation:** The permeation process is done via pores. Pores are made in hydrogels through phase separation during synthesis. The average size of the pore, the size distribution, and interconnections among them are the key factors of a unique hydrogel [5, 6].

6.3   CLASSIFICATION OF HYDROGELS [1, 7–10]

Hydrogels may be classified into different types:

A. Based on source

Hydrogels can be made up of either natural or synthetic or the combination together.

1) *Natural*: Examples includes pectin, agarose, collagen, fibrin, etc.
2) *Synthetic*: Examples include PEG-PLA-PEG, PEG-PLGA-PEG, etc.
3) *Combination of both*: An example is collagen-PEG.

B. Based on the method of polymeric composition

Hydrogels can be prepared from the cross-linking of a single monomer unit or a combination of more than one type of monomer.

1) *Homopolymer gel:* In these hydrogels, only one type of hydrophilic monomer is used for preparation and possesses a cross-linked backbone structure. Examples are polyvinyl pyrrolidone (PVP) and poly (acrylic acid) gels.
2) *Co-polymer gel:* These types of hydrogels are composed of a minimum of two co-monomers species in which at least one is hydrophilic. These types of gels can be prepared to be sensitive to certain stimuli such as pH, light, etc. An example is co-polymerization of itaconic acid with N-vinyl-2-pyrrolidone (NVP) as a monomer and N,N-methylene-bisacrylamide (MBAAm), which gives a pH-sensitive gel.
3) *Interpenetrating polymer network (IPN):* These hydrogels are made up of two polymers formed without covalent bonds but cross-linked among similar molecules. In IPN, the bulk of the matrix, i.e., polymer, acts as a reservoir for the active agent and releases it in a long-term manner. An example is an IFN blend of chitosan and hydroxyethyl cellulose.

C. Based on ionic charges

Hydrogels can be classified into four types based on their ionic charges:

1) *Neutral hydrogel (nonionic)*: These hydrogels do not have any charges. Examples are dextran and agarose.
2) *Anionic hydrogels*: These hydrogels are negatively charged. Examples are pectin and hyaluronic acid.
3) *Cationic hydrogels*: These have positive charges. Examples are polylysine and chitosan.
4) *Ampholytic hydrogels*: These hydrogels have both positive and negative characters. Examples are collagen and fibrin.

6.4   APPLICATIONS

6.4.1   DIAPERS

Highly adsorbent diapers have the characteristics of being waterless or dry even after substantial adsorption of water. Here, the property of hydrogel for water adsorption is being used by multinational companies. These hydrogel-loaded diapers hold water at maximum extent; most of them are fabricated with different concentrations of sodium polyacrylate, which reduces the dermatological problems related to prolonged contact with wet tissues [11, 12].

6.4.2   WATERING BEADS FOR PLANTS

These hydrogels are fabricated not for retaining water but to sustain releasing water. The release of water into plant species is the attractive feature of hydrogels in the market, from horticulture to plant genetic engineering [13].

6.4.3   TISSUE ENGINEERING

Hydrogels can represent the physiochemical and biological properties of most human native tissues and therefore can be applied in tissue engineering as tissue replacements [14, 15]. pH-sensitive gels have been applied to deliver macromolecules into the cellular system and release drugs due to acidic conditions [16]. Such gels change themselves according to the tissues environment.

6.4.4   BIOMEDICAL APPLICATIONS

6.4.4.1   Drug Delivery

Before administration of the hydrogel into the body, it first has to be incorporated with the desired drug or therapeutic agent [17]. This can be done by the two following methods:

1) In the first method, the hydrogel and drug are mixed together, and the polymer is allowed to cross-link. If necessary, initiators and cross-linkers are added. The drug is present within the matrix of the polymerized gel.
2) In the second method, an already polymerized gel is allowed to sit in the drug solution. The drug solution is absorbed into the gel until equilibrium is achieved [18].

After loading the drug, the gel is dried and ready for use.

6.4.4.2   Drug Release Mechanism Using Hydrogels

The hydrophilic nature of hydrogels to imbibe water makes hydrogels an excellent tool in drug delivery systems. Hydrogels have capacity to absorb a huge quantity of water, sometimes even greater than 90% of their own weight. For purposes of drug release using hydrogels, pharmaceutically active agents are encapsulated within hydrogels, and this can be done by physical entrapment, covalent conjugation, or controlled self-assembly. Owed to their rapid and controllable diffusion rate, hydrogels have been considered a promising vehicle for drug delivery systems for diseases such as diabetes, osteoarthritis, cancer therapy, etc. The main advantage of using hydrogels is their drug delivery in a controlled manner for a longer duration, rending the drug active for a longer time [19–21].

6.4.4.3   Delivery of Drug through Hydrogel Occurs Mainly through Three Mechanisms [19, 22]

6.4.4.3.1   Diffusion Controlled Mechanism

This is the most accepted and popular mechanism model for release of drug from hydrogels. This type of diffusion depends on the structure and morphology of the polymer and is based on the concentration gradient of the drug. An example is the release of doxorubicin from pluronic-based hydrogels composed of poly(ethylene glycol) and polyxamer in response to increasing temperature and increasing hydrophobicity [19, 23].

It can be of two types:

6.4.4.3.1.1   Reservoir Device System   In this model, the drug remains at the core of the gel, encapsulated by the polymeric membrane. Drug release via polymeric membrane follows Fick's law of diffusion down the concentration gradient, i.e., from the core of the gel to the surrounding media. To extended drug release at constant rate, the drug is incorporated at a very high concentration at the core [24].

6.4.4.3.1.2   Matrix Device System   In this method, the drug is homogeneously distributed all over the gel and is released through the macromolecular pores in the polymeric hydrogel rather than from the core as in a reservoir device. The release rate is proportional to the square root of time [25].

6.4.4.3.2   Chemically Controlled Mechanism

In this mechanism, drug molecules are released by reversible or irreversible enzymatic and hydrolytic reactions within the matrix, and the amount of drug release at a particular time is dependent on the rate of degradation of bonds. In cases of erodible polymers, the rate depends on the rate of degradation and dissolution of the hydrogel. In hydrophilic polymers, erosion occurs all over the polymeric matrix whereas it takes place only on the polymeric surface in hydrophobic polymers [26]. An example is the release of doxorubicin from degradation of disulfide cross-links in the presence of glutathione tripeptide in cases of poly (oligo(ethylene oxide)-methyl methacrylate) gel.

6.4.4.3.3   Swelling Controlled Mechanism

As the hydrophilic matrix absorbs solvent molecules, the gel swells up and the volume increases, which results in the increase in the size of the pores. As the pore size increases, the drug molecules are released from the polymer. In this case, drug diffusion is faster than hydrogel expansion. An example is the release of hydrophilic doxorubicin molecules from a thermosensitive nanogel during its swelling process. Thermosensitive nanogel undergoes a reversible phase transition changing from hydrophilic (swelling) to hydrophobic (shrinking) as a function of temperature change [27].

6.4.5   Advantages of Hydrogels [28, 29]

- Hydrogels have a high degree of plasticity or flexibility and are a close resemblance to natural tissue due to their significant liquid content.

- The features of hydrogels are controlled by external factors that have the ability to sense changes in pH, temperature, or concentration of metabolite and release drugs accordingly.
- Hydrogels are more patient compliant than injections as they can be taken through parenteral routes.
- Hydrogels are readily transforming.
- Controlled drug release can be achieved using hydrogels to achieve a target delivery with the desired release rate and site.
- They are biocompatible, non-immunogenic, and biodegradable and show minimal toxicity.

6.4.6 Disadvantages of Hydrogels [30]

- Hydrogels are expensive.
- Hydrogels are non-adherent in nature; they may need to be protected by a secondary dressing.
- Hydrogels have low mechanical strength (in many reports).
- They can be hard to load with drugs/nutrients (in some cases).

REFERENCES

[1] E.M. Ahmed, Hydrogel: Preparation, characterization, and applications: A review, *Journal of Advanced Research*, 6 (2015) 105–121.
[2] H. Holback, Y. Yeo, K. Park, 1 — Hydrogel swelling behavior and its biomedical applications, in: S. Rimmer (Ed.) *Biomedical Hydrogels*, Woodhead Publishing, Cambridge, 2011, pp. 3–24.
[3] B.V. Slaughter, S.S. Khurshid, O.Z. Fisher, A. Khademhosseini, N.A. Peppas, Hydrogels in regenerative medicine, *Advanced Materials*, 21 (2009) 3307–3329.
[4] T.L. Porter, R. Stewart, J. Reed, K. Morton, Models of hydrogel swelling with applications to hydration sensing, *Sensors* (Basel), 7 (2007) 1980–1991.
[5] A.S. Hoffman, Hydrogels for biomedical applications, *Advanced Drug Delivery Reviews*, 64 (2012) 18–23.
[6] F. Ganji, F.S. Vasheghani, F.E. Vasheghani, Theoretical description of hydrogel swelling: A review (2010).
[7] F. Ullah, M.B.H. Othman, F. Javed, Z. Ahmad, H.M. Akil, Classification, processing and application of hydrogels: A review, *Materials Science and Engineering: C*, 57 (2015) 414–433.
[8] K. Varaprasad, G.M. Raghavendra, T. Jayaramudu, M.M. Yallapu, R. Sadiku, A mini review on hydrogels classification and recent developments in miscellaneous applications, *Materials Science and Engineering: C*, 79 (2017) 958–971.
[9] R. Singhal, K. Gupta, A review: Tailor-made hydrogel structures (classifications and synthesis parameters), *Polymer-Plastics Technology and Engineering*, 55 (2016) 54–70.
[10] M. Mahinroosta, Z.J. Farsangi, A. Allahverdi, Z. Shakoori, Hydrogels as intelligent materials: A brief review of synthesis, properties and applications, *Materials Today Chemistry*, 8 (2018) 42–55.
[11] P. Chawla, A. Ranjan Srivastava, P. Pandey, V. Chawla, Hydrogels: A journey from diapers to gene delivery, *Mini Reviews in Medicinal Chemistry*, 14 (2014) 154–167.
[12] H. Omidian, K. Park, Introduction to hydrogels, in: *Biomedical Applications of Hydrogels Handbook*, Springer, New York, 2010, pp. 1–16.

[13] B. Azeem, K. KuShaari, Z.B. Man, A. Basit, T.H. Thanh, Review on materials & methods to produce controlled release coated urea fertilizer, *Journal of Controlled Release*, 181 (2014) 11–21.

[14] S. Van Vlierberghe, P. Dubruel, E. Schacht, Biopolymer-based hydrogels as scaffolds for tissue engineering applications: A review, *Biomacromolecules*, 12 (2011) 1387–1408.

[15] B. Dhandayuthapani, Y. Yoshida, T. Maekawa, D.S. Kumar, Polymeric scaffolds in tissue engineering application: A review, *International Journal of Polymer Science*, 2011 (2011).

[16] V. Balamuralidhara, T. Pramodkumar, N. Srujana, M. Venkatesh, N.V. Gupta, K. Krishna, H. Gangadharappa, pH sensitive drug delivery systems: A review, *American Journal of Drug Discovery and Development*, 1 (2011) 25.

[17] M. Hamidi, A. Azadi, P. Rafiei, Hydrogel nanoparticles in drug delivery, *Advanced Drug Delivery Reviews*, 60 (2008) 1638–1649.

[18] T.R. Hoare, D.S. Kohane, Hydrogels in drug delivery: Progress and challenges, *Polymer*, 49 (2008) 1993–2007.

[19] J. Li, D.J. Mooney, Designing hydrogels for controlled drug delivery, *Nature Reviews Materials*, 1 (2016) 16071.

[20] B. Baumann, T. Jungst, S. Stichler, S. Feineis, O. Wiltschka, M. Kuhlmann, M. Lindén, J. Groll, Control of nanoparticle release kinetics from 3D printed hydrogel scaffolds, *Angewandte Chemie International Edition*, 56 (2017) 4623–4628.

[21] D. Caccavo, S. Cascone, G. Lamberti, A.A. Barba, Controlled drug release from hydrogel-based matrices: Experiments and modeling, *International Journal of Pharmaceutics*, 486 (2015) 144–152.

[22] P. Ramburrun, P. Kumar, Y.E. Choonara, L.C. du Toit, V. Pillay, Design and characterization of neurodurable gellan-xanthan pH-responsive hydrogels for controlled drug delivery, *Expert Opinion on Drug Delivery*, 14 (2017) 291–306.

[23] P.I. Lee, Diffusion-controlled matrix systems, in: *Treatise on Controlled Drug Delivery*, Taylor and Francis Routledge, Abingdon, 2017, pp. 155–197.

[24] A. Kumar, J. Pillai, Implantable drug delivery systems: An overview, in: *Nanostructures for the Engineering of Cells, Tissues and Organs*, Elsevier, 2018, pp. 473–511.

[25] E. Caló, V.V. Khutoryanskiy, Biomedical applications of hydrogels: A review of patents and commercial products, *European Polymer Journal*, 65 (2015) 252–267.

[26] M. Rizwan, R. Yahya, A. Hassan, M. Yar, A.D. Azzahari, V. Selvanathan, F. Sonsudin, C.N. Abouloula, pH sensitive hydrogels in drug delivery: Brief history, properties, swelling, and release mechanism, material selection and applications, *Polymers*, 9 (2017) 137.

[27] S. Kim, K. Lee, C. Cha, Refined control of thermoresponsive swelling/deswelling and drug release properties of poly (N-isopropylacrylamide) hydrogels using hydrophilic polymer crosslinkers, *Journal of Biomaterials Science, Polymer Edition*, 27 (2016) 1698–1711.

[28] F. Ketabat, S. Khorshidi, A. Karkhaneh, Application of minimally invasive injectable conductive hydrogels as stimulating scaffolds for myocardial tissue engineering, *Polymer International*, 67 (2018) 975–982.

[29] S.J. Buwalda, T. Vermonden, W.E. Hennink, Hydrogels for therapeutic delivery: Current developments and future directions, *Biomacromolecules*, 18 (2017) 316–330.

[30] T. Billiet, M. Vandenhaute, J. Schelfhout, S. Van Vlierberghe, P. Dubruel, A review of trends and limitations in hydrogel-rapid prototyping for tissue engineering, *Biomaterials*, 33 (2012) 6020–6041.

7 Hydrogels and Their Imaging Application

Darryl Taylor and Rupak Dua

CONTENTS

7.1 INTRODUCTION

Hydrogels refer to a class of polymer materials with hydrophilic properties that can retain large volumes of water while maintaining its general structure [1]. Hydrogel, when exposed to water, can absorb enough water to swell several times its original size. The molecular structure of hydrogels contains a cross-linked polymeric backbone, which prevents the hydrogel from getting dissolved in water, and hydrophilic functional groups that bond to water through hydrogen bonding. Hydrogels are an attractive material to use in practical application in many fields due to their versatility, and they can be classified through their origin, structure, and mechanical properties [2] Figure 7.1 represents the swelling of hydrogels from a dehydrated to a hydrated one.

Hydrogels can have natural or synthetic origins [3]. A typical example of a naturally occurring hydrogel is the protein collagen, which is found in structural components of biological systems [4]. Other examples of natural hydrogels are polysaccharides, such as cellulose and proteins, that are part of the extracellular matrix of the cell, such as fibrin [5]. In practical application, synthetic hydrogels are developed to solve biological, mechanical, and biomedical engineering problems. For instance, a specific hydrogel can be synthesized for adhering to natural tissue or use in drug delivery systems or imaging applications. Each of these applications require hydrogels with different functional properties.

Hydrogel functional properties are expressed through the intermolecular interactions between the hydrophobic and hydrophilic components of its polymeric

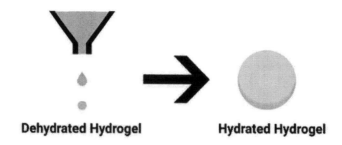

Dehydrated Hydrogel   **Hydrated Hydrogel**

FIGURE 7.1   Pictorial representation of swelling of the hydrogel.

backbone, as well as its structure [6]. Several cross-linking methods are used to control the distribution of water throughout a hydrogel. When a polysaccharide is exposed to gamma-ray radiation, cross-links begin to appear randomly in its structure. These random distributions are then compared with each other, and similar desirable distributions are assimilated to create homogeneous cross-linking patterns within a single synthesized hydrogel [7]. The amount of cross-link patterns is directly proportional to the mechanical strength of the hydrogel. The polymeric backbone of hydrogels is elastic in nature. This elasticity can be characterized by storage modulus and loss modulus, which are functions of cross-linked structures in hydrogels. To model elasticity, modulus functions are employed [8]. These functions have parameters of destiny, temperature, and molecular weight.

Furthermore, hydrogel functional properties depend on the covalent interactions and molecular forces of the polymer or polymers used [9]. The mechanisms of non-covalent interactions within hydrogel structures also strongly contribute to the behavior of hydrogels and hydrogel systems as the behavior of water changes within hydrogel structures. Hydrogels absorb a considerable amount of water [10] and can have up to 99% water content. So, the mechanical and functional properties of water and its behavior need to be considered when developing specific hydrogels.

There are three classifications of water's structure-property relationship with hydrogels: unbound water that does not adhere to the polymer chain, water that is weakly bound to the polymer chain, and bound water [8]. Weakly bound and bound water molecules exhibit different physical behavior than normal water, such as a lower freezing point.

Hydrogels can have pores and microchannels as well [11], although this is different from the porous characteristic of biological tissue like bone. Pores exist in hydrogels due to the motion of backbone polymer chains; this quality is essential for tissue integration [12]. Pores are also useful for mass transfer as drug delivery systems can be readily controlled with porous hydrogel networks. Pores are also crucial for purification processes such as dialysis as hydrogels can be created to force faster mass transfer.

Porous hydrogels can be obtained by 3D (three dimensional) printing polymers [13, 14] or by simply drilling holes. Pores have a direct effect on the mechanical behavior of hydrogels. First, the Young's modulus of the hydrogel increases as porosity increases and mass flux varies with pore size and number. Overall, the mechanical strength of a hydrogel is completely determined by its polymeric backbone [15].

Another essential quality of hydrogels is the rate of swelling and dehydration. When a hydrogel contacts water, the water molecules begin to adhere to the hydrophilic components of the polymer, and as the hydrogel swells, more water is allowed to enter the hydrogel system where the weak bound and bound layers start to appear. This process continues until equilibrium is reached and the hydrogel ceases expansion. The swelling rate of hydrogels can be increased by increasing the number of ionic groups in the polymer backbone. These ions serve to attract more water molecules, which increases the rate of expansion. In short, the more hydrophilic the polymer component of a hydrogel is, the higher its ability to quickly swell [16].

Dehydration occurs through evaporation of bound water molecules by heating. First, the outer layers of water that are weakly bound to the hydrogel begin to evaporate; afterward, the dehydration process is the reverse of the swelling process in that bound water molecules escape the hydrogel and are evaporated away. When a hydrogel is exceptionally dehydrated, it has brittle mechanical behavior similar to glass. The most critical application linked with swelling and dehydration of hydrogel is drug loading into the hydrogel. Drugs can be loaded into hydrogel systems in two ways: either by contact with water with a high concentration of aqueous drugs or conjugate drugs that are captured by the polymeric backbone. However, the latter may have issues with purification and drug transfer. A specific hydrogel system can be manufactured to better transfer drugs throughout a biological system. Other components of drug loading and transfer rate are the intermolecular attractions of the drug itself. Physical properties of the drug such as solubility and molecular size factor into the loading rate of hydrogels [7].

Hydrogels' versatility arises when complicated applications are needed. For example, hydrogels that have the ability to swell quickly may have weak functional properties. To circumvent this a system with multiple hydrogels with different functional properties can be prepared. These systems are created using numerous polymerization techniques where different functional hydrogels are cross-linked together in an efficient ways to solve complex applications [2].

Hydrogels have been used in a wide variety of applications including tissue engineering applications [17–19], fabrication of contact lenses [20], dye and heavy metal ions removal and detection [21], biosensors, pH sensors [22], wound repair [23], management of drug delivery systems [23], etc. In general, hydrogels have a variety of applications in biomedical fields and medicine. Due to their versatility, hydrogel systems have been gaining popularity. Hydrogels with nanocomposite components are formed through physical and chemical cross-linking, which characterize the intrinsic and extrinsic properties of hydrogels. The nanocomposite hydrogels allow for diverse applications in imaging and sensors [24]. The physical and chemical properties of hydrogels can be applied for delivering and targeting desired biological environments in imaging applications. To understand the behavior of hydrogel systems in biological environments, optics are used to image and analyze biochemical processes.

Applied optics in biological applications is an emerging field that uses hydrogels to observe and mimic natural biological systems [25]. In the field of biologically inspired optics, hydrogels can be used to analyze self-assembly processes of cellular systems and the interactions of nanofibers and as biosensors to identify tissue deformations to classify tumors [19]. Many applications of hydrogel networks and optical imaging techniques have extensive application in detecting tumors and other undesirable physiological signals and in drug delivery. The powerful potential of using hydrogel networks comes from the versatility of hydrogels to incorporate components that allow for faster signal detection and drug delivery and efficiency in biological environments. To this end, the purpose of this chapter is to provide the use of hydrogels for imaging application in biological systems and offer our perspective on their future use.

7.2 IMAGING APPLICATIONS

7.2.1 DRUG DELIVERY

The imaging applications of hydrogels can be applied to drug delivery systems. The monitoring and tracking of drug agents are important features of an effective hydrogel system [21]. To create more efficient hydrogel systems that report changes in drug distribution, several methods have been implemented. One of the ways introduces a metal chelator, which is a metal atom ionically bonded to a single central atom [26]. These metal ions are used to detect other inorganic ions such as heavy metals but can also be used to identify changes in the physical characteristics of cellular environments based on the concentration of the metal chelators. For instance, hydrogels can be utilized to detect not only inorganic ions but also metallic ions such as silver ions using the luminescent Carbon Quantum Dot hydrogels (CQDGs). These hydrogels also improve the fluorescence contrast and selectivity of silver ions [21]. While this addition to the polymeric matrix of a hydrogel does increase signal enhancement, metal ions can be toxic as the toxicity of the metal can warp peptide interactions.

Being non-toxic and biological compatible, another imaging application of such hydrogel systems is to image enhanced drug delivery systems via MRI-based theranostic filament hydrogels (Figure 7.2). Responsive components of hydrogel systems have also been utilized to combine drug delivery systems and imaging techniques [19]. MRI systems can adhere to hydrogel networks, creating stricter functional parameters such as magnetic targeting, contrast enhancement, and controlled swelling and shrinking through heat conduction and induction.

7.2.2 DIAGNOSTIC IMAGING

To effectively target specific tissues, cross-linked hydrogel structures have been examined as a solution to drug delivery challenges in medical fields. The functional characteristics and properties, such as delivery effectiveness, size, shape, and composition of hydrogels used for diagnostic imaging, take advantage of different properties of hydrogel networks based on the type of imaging used. For diagnostic imaging, the chemical and mechanical flexibility and the degree of cross-linking of hydrogel matrices must be considered to create desirable hydrogel systems that transport different drug substituents. Imaging modalities, including magnetic resonance imaging, positron emission tomography, single-photon emission computed tomography, ultrasound imaging, and fluorescent imaging, are used in medicine to detect the operation of hydrogel network functionality.

MR imaging has continuous use in imaging fields due to its ability, with the addition of contrast elements like iron oxide and gadolinium, to sharply image soft tissue [27] and is primarily used to analyze the behavior of nanoparticles in different soft tissue environments (Figure 7.3).

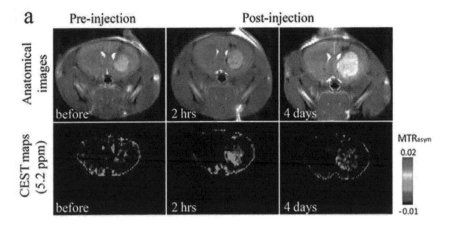

FIGURE 7.2   MRI images showing brain tumors at different time points with respect to the time of injection of the nanofiber hydrogel.

Source: Adopted and with copyright permission from ACS nano [19].

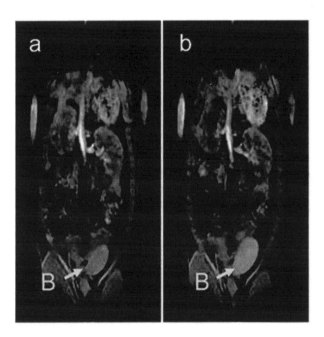

FIGURE 7.3   Images of rat (a) before and (b) one hour after an injection of contrast element gadolinium, GadoSiPEG2C, that accumulated in the bladder (B) and made it brighter.

Source: Adopted and with copyright permission from the *Journal of the American Chemical Society* [27].

However, iron oxides have low sensitivity, so large amounts of the agent must be used to produce high contrast images [28]. A solution to this problem employs iron oxide nanocrystals, which have been shown to have a similar contrasting effect when compared to nanoparticles [29]. There has been the development of hydrogel hybridized with iron oxides for MRI and drug delivery applications. Recently, a research group led by Zhang developed hyaluronic acid nanogels hybridized with iron oxide nanoparticles. The hydrogel encapsulates these iron oxide particles and acts as a carrier; due to their degradation by the hyaluronidase present in the body, it releases iron oxides nanoparticles, thus allowing the utilization of imaging agents as tracers of the hydrogel degradation using MRI [30]. This method of imaging is used for detecting changes in tissue environments and tumors or any other changes that may affect the behavior of observed environments.

Positron emission tomography (PET), which uses emitted gamma rays from radioactive ions, has a low spatial resolution, and contrast agents are not easily obtained or synthesized. However, because of its high sensitivity, it is used for detection applications. It has been shown that PET integrated hydrogels can be used to detect the accumulation and consumption of nanoparticles like drugs and other macromolecules in biological environments [31].

7.2.3 Tumor Detection

Recently, an increase in desirability for materials with unique features and applications in medicine has led to the development of hydrogel technology that fits emerging needs, especially for the detection of malignant cancer cells [32]. There are several categories of imaging that can be applied to hydrogel systems, and each class refers to the purpose of the hydrogel system's detection abilities. For example, a process referred to as elasticity imaging employs techniques that ultrasonically image soft tissue while applying compressive loads to hydrogel systems and uses these images to obtain maps of disease patterns that have links to breast tumor growth [33].

Endoscopic molecular imaging (EMI) can selectively detect tumors while being minimally non-invasive. Hydrogel networks can be used for EMI applications to detect tumors that are difficult to detect and image. Endoscopic molecular imaging that employs hydrogel is formed through self-assembly processes that create hydrogels to enhance the understanding of tumor formations and pathways dependent imaging. These systems can operate in cellular environments while maintaining a highly ordered structure and respond quickly to physiological signals linked to malignant tumors [19]. Another approach is self-assembly process for fabrication of self-assemble biocatalytic, which uses an enzyme sensitive group to self-assemble into nanofibers that generate more complex detection networks.

Malignant cancer cells and metastasis are associated with altered signals from biomolecules like proteins and glycans [34]. These signals are currently being analyzed using detection techniques that involve different imaging operations such as MRI and EMI. The characteristics of self-assembly dependent imaging are the shifts observed for different molecular networks, which dramatically influence the contrast in fluorescent imaging. The self-assembly process is necessary from a design perspective as the efficiency of the desired drug and the response time to changes in the environment overall improve the functionality of hydrogels [35].

7.2.4 INTRACELLULAR IMAGING

Hydrogel networks are not limited to detecting tumors and delivering drugs to targeted tissues but also are used for data analysis of biological networks within the human body [36]. The optical sensing capabilities of hydrogels for monitoring chemical changes in blood and bioreactor fluids are useful in many biomedical applications [37]. The research group led by Wu and Zhou categorized hydrogel network probes that are used in medicine. A Type 1 probe utilized antibodies to detect drugs and other complex macromolecules and their specific protein and nucleotide sequences in a mixture. Another type of probe, Type 2, utilized the optical properties of a hydrogel network and its reaction to desirable substances and is used to detect pH fluctuations [38]. Metallic components are integrated into the hydrogel polymer network, and these metallic ions serve to create an ion gradient that changes based on the difference in pH. Further, fluorescent compounds are used along with this gradient to analyze pH change qualitatively (Figure 7.4) [39]. The last classification of probes, Type 3, used the polymer components of hydrogels to detect changes in chemical signals and other physical characteristics of biological environments such as pH, temperature, and sugar concentrations.

In medicine, these probes can be applied in detecting and accurately diagnosing diseases that are linked to chemical and physical changes in intracellular

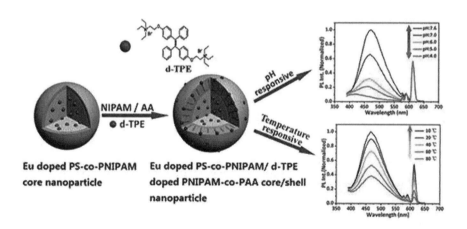

FIGURE 7.4 Scheme showing the designing of a dual-emissive hydrogel particle system comprised of polymers N-isopropylacrylamide (NIPAM) and acrylic acid (AA) that provides photoluminescence response to pH and temperature [39].

Source: Adopted and with copyright permission from ACS nano.

environments. Type 3 detection networks undergo chemical and conformational changes to external stimulation, leading the physical characteristics of the hydrogel probe to alter as well.

To properly integrate optical and polymeric components of hydrogel probes, dye molecules and other fluorescents are introduced to the hydrogel network through absorption or integration. Each probe classification depends on the type of dye molecule introduced and the method in which they permeate through the hydrogel network. In general, dye molecules are generally used to produce Type 2 probes whereas organic fluorescent molecules are used to synthesize Type 3 probes. Type 1 probes are generated using quantum dot integration methods.

Intracellular hydrogel networks are used to monitor changes in pH, temperature, glucose concentration, and common biological ions. Each classification of the probe is used for different detection apparatuses. Type 2 probes have been implemented to detect changes in metallic ions like potassium, chlorine, magnesium, and calcium. Type 3 probes detect temperature and pH in living cellular environments and relate temperature change with change in a cellular environment [38].

7.2.5 TISSUE ENGINEERING IMAGING

Tissue engineering combines bioengineering, biology, and mechanics to create functionally integrated tissue that serves to repair or replace damaged tissue or organs [40]. Engineered scaffolds composed of hydrogels have been reported useful for bone and cartilage tissue engineering [17, 18] because of their similarity to the properties of native cartilage and bone tissue [41].

The migration of cells from engineered tissues to native tissue is one of the characteristics of engineered tissue. To further understand this behavior, hydrogel networks that are integrated into cartilage and bone scaffolds must have imaging components as well. Cell movement and protein generation in 3D environments can be captured by hydrogel systems that have fluorescent markers on the desired protein. However, this method has issues when applied to multicellular environments. For example, the difference in size and mechanical behavior of individual cells in multicellular environments makes it difficult to design a hydrogel network as it is

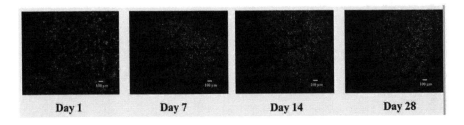

FIGURE 7.5   Images showing the viability of chondrocytes in hydrogel over a period of 28 days for their application in tissue-engineered cartilage [18].

Source: Adopted from PLOS ONE under Creative Commons Attribution License. [18].

difficult to predict how hydrogel networks will interact with many cells at the same instance [41].

7.2.6 BIOSENSORS

Another category of hydrogel used for imaging applications includes biosensors [42]. The imaging biosensors are analyzed based on adsorption rate and inhibitions or catalyzation of biochemical reactions. The use of hydrogels for creating efficient and durable biosensors is vital for distinguishing not only the concentration of specific proteins and other biological macromolecules but also for classifying biomolecular interactions [24]. The extracellular matrix (ECM) of a cell is mimicked in tissue engineering to create engineered tissue or material that serves to replace and repair native soft tissues [35]. While these processes are reproducible, there is a lack of analytical information on the behavior and biodegradation of engineered tissue and material after integration [33]. One of the methods of analyzing the behavior of integrated hydrogel biomaterial is diamagnetic chemical exchange saturation transfer (CEST) magnetic resonance [35]. CEST magnetic resonance was used to analyze the distribution of an ECM hydrogel as it operates in a biological environment. CEST is used to selectively visualize the distribution of diffusion through hydrogels of specific proteins and metabolization processes in animal models. This process is for the purpose of analyzing the ability of engineered biomaterial to mimic and facilitate the repair of native tissue [19].

TABLE 7.1
Summary of Application of Hydrogels in Imaging for Biological Systems [17–19, 21, 24, 31, 33, 35, 38, 41]

Application of hydrogels	Target area	Techniques
Drug delivery	Cellular environments	• Metal chelator • Carbon Quantum Dot hydrogels • MRI-based theranostic filament
Diagnostic imaging	Soft tissues	Hydrogels integrated with imaging modalities including magnetic resonance imaging, positron emission tomography, single-photon emission computed tomography, ultrasound imaging, and fluorescent imaging
Tumor detection	Areas difficult to detect through conventional methods	• Elasticity imaging • Endoscopic molecular imaging
Intracellular imaging	Intracellular matrix	Hydrogel network probes
Tissue engineering	Soft and hard tissues	• Scaffolding • Integrating fluorescent markers in hydrogels

7.3   CURRENT AND FUTURE OUTLOOK

A summary of the hydrogels that are used imaging applications for diagnostics and therapeutics presented in this chapter has been shown in Table 7.1. Ultimately, providing a hydrogel network with imaging enhancement using fluorescent probes or any other approach would be beneficial for many areas in medical science. Further, optically stimulated molecules within the hydrogel would be of great benefit to quickly diagnose various diseases. Tissue engineering, in particular, is a significant component of hydrogel network applications as understanding the process between integrating engineered tissue and native tissue is of extreme importance to tissue engineering applications. Currently, there is not much information available about the migration of cells from engineered tissue to native tissue in tissue engineering applications. Hydrogel networks that can image the configuration and migration of engineered cells would be useful for developing engineered tissue that will integrate more readily to native tissue. Musculoskeletal system diseases could also be better understood and detected by hydrogel network imaging. In addition, hydrogels with imaging modularity could be used in additive manufacturing technology to create 3D printed organs and tissues. Self-healing hydrogels with optical capabilities would be able to repair wounds as well as monitor the changes of the degradable biomaterial.

7.4   CONCLUSIONS

The potential benefits of the use of the hydrogels in imaging applications in diagnostics and therapeutics are promising. In recent years, much research has been done on hydrogels for imaging applications in various biological domains, including drug delivery, chemical and biological signal sensors, tissue engineering, and tumor detection. Renewed interest in this area may provide the necessary breakthrough in enhancing hydrogel networks with more advanced imaging capabilities and, in doing so, moving from benchtop and in vivo studies to functional assessment in clinical trials over the next decade, thus opening great possibilities in the future.

REFERENCES

[1]   E. Caló, V.V. Khutoryanskiy, Biomedical applications of hydrogels: A review of patents and commercial products, *European Polymer Journal*, 65 (2015) 252–267.
[2]   E.M. Ahmed, Hydrogel: Preparation, characterization, and applications: A review, *Journal of Advanced Research*, 6 (2015) 105–121.
[3]   M. Hamidi, A. Azadi, P. Rafiei, Hydrogel nanoparticles in drug delivery, *Advanced Drug Delivery Reviews*, 60 (2008) 1638–1649.
[4]   Y. Hu, H. Wang, J. Wang, S. Wang, W. Liao, Y. Yang, Y. Zhang, D. Kong, Z. Yang, Supramolecular hydrogels inspired by collagen for tissue engineering, *Organic & Biomolecular Chemistry*, 8 (2010) 3267–3271.
[5]   J. Zhu, R.E. Marchant, Design properties of hydrogel tissue-engineering scaffolds, *Expert Review of Medical Devices*, 8 (2011) 607–626.
[6]   Q. Chai, Y. Jiao, X. Yu, Hydrogels for biomedical applications: Their characteristics and the mechanisms behind them, *Gels*, 3 (2017) 6.
[7]   V. Gun'ko, I. Savina, S. Mikhalovsky, Properties of water bound in hydrogels, *Gels*, 3 (2017) 37.

[8] L.J. Dooling, D.A. Tirrell, Engineering the dynamic properties of protein networks through sequence variation, *ACS Central Science*, 2 (2016) 812–819.

[9] A.S. Hoffman, Hydrogels for biomedical applications, *Advanced Drug Delivery Reviews*, 64 (2012) 18–23.

[10] N. Peppas, P. Bures, W. Leobandung, H. Ichikawa, Hydrogels in pharmaceutical formulations, *European Journal of Pharmaceutics and Biopharmaceutics*, 50 (2000) 27–46.

[11] L. Bosio, G. Johari, M. Oumezzine, J. Teixeira, X-ray and neutron scattering studies of the structure of water in a hydrogel, *Chemical Physics Letters*, 188 (1992) 113–118.

[12] I.M. El-Sherbiny, M.H. Yacoub, Hydrogel scaffolds for tissue engineering: Progress and challenges, *Global Cardiology Science and Practice* (2013) 38.

[13] D.M. Kirchmajer, R. Gorkin Iii, An overview of the suitability of hydrogel-forming polymers for extrusion-based 3D-printing, *Journal of Materials Chemistry B*, 3 (2015) 4105–4117.

[14] Y. Zhao, B. Liu, L. Pan, G. Yu, 3D nanostructured conductive polymer hydrogels for high-performance electrochemical devices, *Energy & Environmental Science*, 6 (2013) 2856–2870.

[15] Y-C. Chiu, S. Kocagöz, J.C. Larson, E.M. Brey, Evaluation of physical and mechanical properties of porous poly (ethylene glycol)-co-(l-lactic acid) hydrogels during degradation, *PLoS One*, 8 (2013) e60728.

[16] R. Parhi, Cross-linked hydrogel for pharmaceutical applications: A review, *Advanced Pharmaceutical Bulletin*, 7 (2017) 515–530.

[17] R. Dua, J. Centeno, S. Ramaswamy, Augmentation of engineered cartilage to bone integration using hydroxyapatite, *Journal of Biomedical Materials Research Part B: Applied Biomaterials*, 102 (2014) 922–932.

[18] R. Dua, K. Comella, R. Butler, G. Castellanos, B. Brazille, A. Claude, A. Agarwal, J. Liao, S. Ramaswamy, Integration of stem cell to chondrocyte-derived cartilage matrix in healthy and osteoarthritic states in the presence of hydroxyapatite nanoparticles, *PLoS One*, 11 (2016) e0149121.

[19] L.L. Lock, Y. Li, X. Mao, H. Chen, V. Staedtke, R. Bai, W. Ma, R. Lin, Y. Li, G. Liu, H. Cui, One-component supramolecular filament hydrogels as theranostic label-free magnetic resonance imaging agents, *ACS Nano*, 11 (2017) 797–805.

[20] J. Kopecek, Hydrogels: From soft contact lenses and implants to self-assembled nanomaterials, *Journal of Polymer Science Part A: Polymer Chemistry*, 47 (2009) 5929–5946.

[21] A. Cayuela, M.L. Soriano, S.R. Kennedy, J. Steed, M. Valcárcel, Fluorescent carbon quantum dot hydrogels for direct determination of silver ions, *Talanta*, 151 (2016) 100–105.

[22] O. Andersson, A. Larsson, T. Ekblad, B. Liedberg, Gradient hydrogel matrix for microarray and biosensor applications: An imaging SPR study, *Biomacromolecules*, 10 (2008) 142–148.

[23] R. Dimatteo, N.J. Darling, T. Segura, In situ forming injectable hydrogels for drug delivery and wound repair, *Advanced Drug Delivery Reviews*, 127 (2018) 167–184.

[24] A. Vashist, A. Kaushik, A. Ghosal, J. Bala, R. Nikkhah-Moshaie, W.A. Wani, P. Manickam, M. Nair, Nanocomposite hydrogels: Advances in nanofillers used for nanomedicine, *Gels*, 4 (2018).

[25] L.P. Lee, R. Szema, Inspirations from biological optics for advanced photonic systems, *Science*, 310 (2005) 1148–1150.

[26] S. Maity, N. Parshi, C. Prodhan, K. Chaudhuri, J. Ganguly, Characterization of a fluorescent hydrogel synthesized using chitosan, polyvinyl alcohol and 9-anthraldehyde for the selective detection and discrimination of trace Fe(3+) and Fe(2+) in water for live-cell imaging, *Carbohydrate Polymers*, 193 (2018) 119–128.

[27] J.L. Bridot, A.C. Faure, S. Laurent, C. Riviere, C. Billotey, B. Hiba, M. Janier, V. Josserand, J.L. Coll, L.V. Elst, R. Muller, S. Roux, P. Perriat, O. Tillement, Hybrid gadolinium oxide nanoparticles: Multimodal contrast agents for in vivo imaging, *Journal of the American Chemical Society*, 129 (2007) 5076–5084.

[28] R.S. Chaughule, S. Purushotham, R.V. Ramanujan, Magnetic nanoparticles as contrast agents for magnetic resonance imaging, *Proceedings of the National Academy of Sciences, India Section A: Physical Sciences*, 82 (2012) 257–268.

[29] N. Lee, T. Hyeon, Designed synthesis of uniformly sized iron oxide nanoparticles for efficient magnetic resonance imaging contrast agents, *Chemical Society Reviews*, 41 (2012) 2575–2589.

[30] Y. Zhang, Y. Sun, X. Yang, J. Hilborn, A. Heerschap, D.A. Ossipov, Injectable in situ forming hybrid iron oxide-hyaluronic acid hydrogel for magnetic resonance imaging and drug delivery, *Macromolecular Bioscience*, 14 (2014) 1249–1259.

[31] D.A. Canelas, K.P. Herlihy, J.M. DeSimone, Top-down particle fabrication: Control of size and shape for diagnostic imaging and drug delivery, *Wiley Interdisciplinary Reviews: Nanomedicine and Nanobiotechnology*, 1 (2009) 391–404.

[32] Y. Kuang, J. Shi, J. Li, D. Yuan, K.A. Alberti, Q. Xu, B. Xu, Pericellular hydrogel/nanonets inhibit cancer cells, *Angewandte Chemie* (International ed. in English), 53 (2014) 8104–8107.

[33] S. Kalyanam, R.D. Yapp, M.F. Insana, Poro-viscoelastic behavior of gelatin hydrogels under compression-implications for bioelasticity imaging, *Journal of Biomechanical Engineering*, 131 (2009) 081005.

[34] J. Lux, A.G. White, M. Chan, C.J. Anderson, A. Almutairi, Nanogels from metal-chelating crosslinkers as versatile platforms applied to copper-64 PET imaging of tumors and metastases, *Theranostics*, 5 (2015) 277–288.

[35] T. Jin, F.J. Nicholls, W.R. Crum, H. Ghuman, S.F. Badylak, M. Modo, Diamagnetic chemical exchange saturation transfer (diaCEST) affords magnetic resonance imaging of extracellular matrix hydrogel implantation in a rat model of stroke, *Biomaterials*, 113 (2017) 176–190.

[36] N.A. Peppas, J.Z. Hilt, A. Khademhosseini, R. Langer, Hydrogels in biology and medicine: From molecular principles to bionanotechnology, *Advanced Materials*, 18 (2006) 1345–1360.

[37] A. Richter, G. Paschew, S. Klatt, J. Lienig, K.F. Arndt, H.P. Adler, Review on hydrogel-based pH sensors and microsensors, *Sensors* (Basel, Switzerland), 8 (2008) 561–581.

[38] W. Wu, S. Zhou, Hybrid micro-/nanogels for optical sensing and intracellular imaging, *Nano Reviews*, 1 (2010).

[39] Y. Zhao, C. Shi, X. Yang, B. Shen, Y. Sun, Y. Chen, X. Xu, H. Sun, K. Yu, B. Yang, Q. Lin, pH- and temperature-sensitive hydrogel nanoparticles with dual photoluminescence for bioprobes, *ACS Nano*, 10 (2016) 5856–5863.

[40] D.S. Benoit, M.P. Schwartz, A.R. Durney, K.S. Anseth, Small functional groups for controlled differentiation of hydrogel-encapsulated human mesenchymal stem cells, *Nature Materials*, 7 (2008) 816–823.

[41] M. Liu, X. Zeng, C. Ma, H. Yi, Z. Ali, X. Mou, S. Li, Y. Deng, N. He, Injectable hydrogels for cartilage and bone tissue engineering, *Bone Research*, 5 (2017) 17014.

[42] D.A. Stenger, G.W. Gross, E.W. Keefer, K.M. Shaffer, J.D. Andreadis, W. Ma, J.J. Pancrazio, Detection of physiologically active compounds using cell-based biosensors, *Trends in Biotechnology*, 19 (2001) 304–309.

8 Hydrogels in Tissue Engineering

Tanya Chhibber, Ravikumar Shinde, Behnaz Lahooti, Sounak Bagchi, Sree Pooja Varahachalam, Anusha Gaddam, Amit K. Jaiswal, Evelyn Gracia, Hitendra S. Chand, Ajeet Kaushik, and Rahul Dev Jayant

CONTENTS

8.1 INTRODUCTION

Tissue engineering is a fast-emerging multidisciplinary field where the principles of biological sciences and bioengineering (i.e. material science, polymer chemistry, cell biology, and tissue transplantation) are used together for the creation of new three-dimensional (3D) biological substitutes that mimic the design of human tissue so that their functions can be improved, restored, or maintained [1, 2]. Tissue engineering has transformed the therapeutic approach in tissue regeneration and replacement, with the goal of overcoming the severity of the shortage of organ donors, by fabricating the functional tissues. The latest development in this area comes from regenerative medicine, in addition to the high demand for tissues and organs needed for transplants [3]. The tissue engineering archetype involves segregation of specific cells via a small biopsy from patients, growing them on a 3D biomimetic scaffold under accurately controlled culture conditions, transporting the structure to the anticipated site in the patient's body, and assisting in new tissue formation onto the scaffold that degrades biologically over time [4].

Several strategies are currently in use to engineering tissues depending on the material scaffolds. These scaffolds act as a synthetic extracellular matrix (ECM) to establish cells into a 3D construction to present stimuli, which leads to the growth and proliferation of preferred tissue [5]. Presently, tissue engineering methods are classified into two essential categories: cell based and scaffold based. The typical tissue engineering method tries to generate an engineered tissue structure by combining cells with a natural or synthetic scaffold matter under favorable culture conditions. The scaffold-based tissue engineering method is more inclined to body's natural capability to regenerate for proper alignment and way of new tissue ingrowth [6]. Figure 8.1 highlights the progress of tissue engineering with regard to

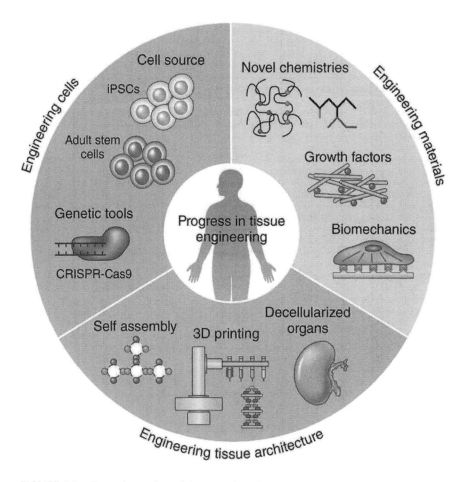

FIGURE 8.1   General overview of tissue engineering.

Source: [7].

the development of cell types used, materials advancement using novel chemistries, and tissue architecture used to improve structural or functional resemblance to the body's tissues [7, 8].

8.2   IMPORTANCE OF TISSUE ENGINEERING

Daily, thousands of surgical operations are performed to substitute or repair tissue that has been impaired via disease or trauma. Tissue engineering aims to play a vital role in regenerating damaged tissue by combining body cells with highly porous scaffold biomaterials [9]. Data obtained from Organ Procurement and Transplant Network (OPTN), showed only 34,769 transplants were performed out of 115,000 patients until January 2018 [10]. The rising trend of increased life expectancy, as well as critical limitations in the use of allogeneic, autologous, and xenogeneic grafts, has kindled scientists around the world to join the quest for new alternative tissue substitutes with unique features for use in tissue engineering [11].

Treatment of damaged tissue emphasizes transplanting tissue from one part of the body to another in the same patient (autograft) or from one individual to another (allograft). Autologous transplantation is hindered because of donor site morbidity and infection or pain in patients due to secondary surgery. Alternative tissue sources from other humans and animals appeared to be challenging mostly because of immunogenic responses by the patients upon implantation and scarcity of donor organs [4]. Scientists and surgeons are opting for tissue engineering to regenerate tissues instead of using transplantation. Tissue engineering has opened a new pathway for treating patients in a minimally invasive and less painful way [4]. Biodegradable synthetic polymers have several advantages over other materials for generating scaffolds in tissue engineering. The essential benefits include the capability to modify mechanical properties and degradation kinetics to match diverse applications. Synthetic polymers are also appealing because they can be modified into different shapes with the desired morphological characteristics favoring tissue ingrowth [12].

8.3   TYPES OF BIOMATERIALS USED FOR TISSUE ENGINEERING

The European Society for Biomaterials (ESB) currently defines biomaterials as "material intended to interface with biological systems to evaluate, treat, augment or replace any tissue, organ or function of the body" [9]. The critical feature that distinguishes biomaterials from other materials is their capability to coexist and interrelate in the presence of tissues or biological systems such as blood, interstitial fluids, immune cells, and molecules without causing an unbearable amount of impairment [3]. The three conventional categories of biodegradable polymers are synthetic, natural, and hybrid materials. In recent years, these have been getting attention due to their excellent features in regenerative remedies [13]. Extensive varieties of natural and synthetically derived polymers are capable of enduring decay; conversely, synthetic biodegradable polymers have been found to have more adaptable and varied biomedical functions, possibly because of more facile capability to undergo tailorable designs and chemical alterations [13].

Naturally occurring biomaterials (chitosan, collagen, alginate, hyaluronic acid, etc.) are extensively used due to biocompatibility and biodegradability. Degradation of biomaterials is one of the significant aspects of naturally occurring polymers. These biomaterials have excellent biocompatibility and growth response due to their presence in an extracellular matrix. Collagen is one of the most extensively used natural biomaterials as scaffolds in diverse biomedical applications [10].

Agarose is another natural polysaccharide possessing distinctive features, which makes it a suitable applicant for tissue engineering. Significant features of agarose such as its excellent thermo-reversible gelation behavior, biocompatibility, and physicochemical characteristics make it an excellent option as a biomaterial for cell growth and controlled or localized delivery of drugs. Agarose is very similar in respect to extracellular matrix, which can be beneficial in the field of tissue engineering [14]. Alginate has been used widely in hydrogels for cell encapsulation, drug delivery, and tissue engineering applications [6]. Polymers, in comparison to metallic and inorganic materials, are suitable applicants for tissue engineering applications due to their excellent physical properties such as low density, easy modification, controlled degradability, and minimal environmental or immunogenic effects [15]. Even though natural polymers have several advantages, there are some disadvantages like not being available in bulk quantities, high cost, and complicated processes to generate scaffolds into specific shapes [13].

Due to some limitations of natural polymers, scientists developed synthetic or semi-synthetic polymers. The most widely used synthetic polymers for drug delivery and tissue engineering purposes are poly (lactic acid) (PLA) [14], poly (glycolic acid) (PGA), poly (lactic-co-glycolide) (PLGA), poly (ε-caprolactone) (PCL), poly (p-dioxanone), etc. [13]. There are non-degradable synthetic biomaterials which are widely used as well, like polyethylene derivatives, poly (methyl) acrylates, poly (tetrafluoroethylene), polyethers, polyacrylamides, polysiloxanes, polyurethanes, etc. These polymers prove advantageous in several ways like reproducible quality, non-immunogenic, and tailored mechanical properties and shapes [10].

Bioactive glasses are structurally brittle but have many desirable features to emphasize ionic release with osteogenic potential, controllable degradation rate, good binding affinity to bone, and capability of becoming hydroxyapatite-like material. Since the arrival of silicate-based 45S5 glass, numerous other formulations have been developed and utilized in bone tissue engineering research [16]. Bioceramics (e.g. calcium phosphate ceramics) are another class of material which also possesses biopolymer-like properties, e.g. integrally tough and slow degrading. They are generally combined with other biodegradable polymers to yield better structures. The most widely used calcium phosphate ceramics are β-tricalcium phosphate (TCP), hydroxyapatite (HA), and biphasic calcium phosphate (BCP), a combination of the previous two matters [16]. Composites are constructed with the aim of combining key features from at least two types of materials. Natural or synthetic polymers are often mixed with inorganic matters to form CaPs or bioglasses [16].

Conducting polymers (CPs) are new generation organic materials that display electrical and optical properties like metals and inorganic semiconductors. CP can be synthesized easily and is flexible during processing. It has enhanced mechanical compatibility and structural tunability with biological cells and organs in comparison to normal electronic inorganic and metal materials. Commonly used CPs are polypyrrole (PPY), polyaniline (PANI), and polythiophene and their derivatives [17]. In contrast, CPs also have issues of poor solubility, non-biodegradability, and chronic inflammation. Aniline oligomers can overcome the issues mentioned prior, as they have good solubility, biocompatibility, and electroactivity, making them outstanding applicants for scaffolds used in tissue engineering. Bioconductive polymers like aniline oligomers display realistic functions for the treatment of different organs or tissues [18].

8.4   HYDROGELS

Hydrogels are three-dimensional network systems composed of two or more components of polymer chains and water that fill the space between macromolecules. Due to their ability to absorb a large amount of water, they become swollen without being dissolved. The hydrophilic nature of hydrogels can be attributed to amino, amide, hydroxyl, and carboxyl moieties present in the polymers. These properties have made them popular in biomedical fields such as drug delivery and tissue engineering [15, 19]. The crosslinking of polymers in hydrogels helps form a 3D network, making them ideal for holding as well as releasing biological molecules in a tailored fashion. The swelling properties and viscoelastic nature of hydrogels can simulate the environment of soft tissue more than any other materials. In addition, they have low interfacial tension and high permeability to biomolecules [5, 20–24]. The porous structure of hydrogels enables the transfer of low molecular weight nutrients and cellular waste, which is vital for cellular viability. In addition, biocompatible and biodegradable hydrogels can direct the migration, growth, and arrangement of cells during cartilage regeneration [25].

8.4.1   MATERIALS USED FOR HYDROGEL PREPARATION

Different materials are used for the preparation of hydrogels, and several more are being studied for their potential application in tissue engineering. The hydrogel scaffolds are produced from various synthetic polymers, e.g. polyethylene glycol, polyethylene oxide, polyvinyl alcohol, polyacrylamide, polyacrylic acid, polypropylene fumarate-co-ethylene glycol, polypeptides polydimethylsiloxane, and natural polymers, e.g. collagen, fibrin, gelatin, alginate, hyaluronic acid, and chitosan [25]. Table 8.1 and Table 8.2 highlight the various natural and synthetic polymers used in hydrogel preparation and their application for tissue regeneration.

8.4.2   TYPES OF HYDROGELS IN TISSUE ENGINEERING

A) **Hybrid hydrogels:** Most of these traditional hydrogel materials have shown promise in tissue engineering; however, it would be unwise to ignore issues like bioactivities, mechanical strength, and degradation kinetics. The limitations of natural materials are due to their immunogenic properties and comparatively poor mechanical strength. Although synthetic polymers can be manufactured at a large scale and are easy to manipulate, most of them work as a passive scaffold only. The synthetic polymers alone usually do

TABLE 8.1

Types of Natural Polymers Used in Hydrogel Preparation and Their Application in Tissues Engineering

		Natural materials			
Sr. no	Polymer	Crosslinking method	Types of cells used	Developed tissue	Reference
1	Hyaluronic acid	Protein interaction and amphiphilic block polymers	Fibroblasts	Connective tissue	Shu et al. 2004
		PEG-derivative crosslinker	Human dermal fibroblasts	Skin	Ghosh et al. 2006
2	Alginate-HA	Chemical crosslinking 2-chloro-1-methylpyridinium iodide and 1,3-diaminopropane	Human hepatocytes	Cardiovascular	Magnani et al. 2000
3	Alginate	By ionic interactions of CaCl2	Chondrocytes	Cartilage	Yamaoka et al. 2006
4	Chitosan-PVA	Chemical crosslinking	Osteoblasts	Bone	Pineda-Castillo et al. 2018
5	Gelatin	Crosslinking with hydrogenation	Hepatocytes	Vascular	Tabata et al. 1994
6	Albumin	Crosslinking using enzymes	Mesenchymal stem cells	Skin	Li et al. 2014
		Crosslinking using enzymes	Myocytes	Cardiac tissue	Amdursky et al. 2018
7	Chitosan	Photo-crosslinked	Mesenchymal stem cells	Bone	Cao et al. 2014
8	Dextran	Dextran-PEG crosslinking	Chondrogenic cells	Cartilage tissue	Jukes et al. 2010
9	Gelatin	Photo-crosslinked	HaCaT	Epidermal tissue	Zhao et al. 2016

not support cellular interactions [26–28]. Combinations of different natural and synthetic polymers can be used to manufacture various hybrid hydrogels. Depending upon the requirements and properties of polymers, the combinations, e.g. PEG, can be used to modify different natural polymers such as dextran, HA, and albumin [28–31].

B) **Interpenetrating and semi-interpenetrating hydrogels:** Hybrid hydrogels are not just limited to combinations of different polymers and are being continuously explored for newer possibilities. The multicomponent hydrogels' ability to form interpenetrating and semi-interpenetrating hydrogels has offered many advantages, such as their characteristic microstructure and mechanical properties, over traditional hydrogels [32]. The hydrogels of gelatin and dextran were functionalized with methacrylate and aldehyde,

TABLE 8.2

Types of Synthetic Polymers Used in Hydrogel Preparation and Their Application in Tissues Engineering

		Synthetic materials			
Sr. no.	Polymer	Crosslinking method	Types of cells used	Developed tissue	Reference
1	PEG	Photo-crosslinked	Chondrocytes	Cartilage	Bryant et al. 2004
		Photo-crosslinked	Islets of Langerhans	Pancreatic	Sawhney et al. 1994
2	PEG-PLA	Photo-crosslinked	Osteoblast	Bone	Burdick and Kristi 2002
		Protein interaction	Islets of Langerhans	Pancreatic	Li and Guan 2011
3	PCL and PLGA	Thermal melting and chemical crosslinkers	hPDLSC	Alveolar bone	Peng et al. 2018
4	PEG-PLA-PVA	Photo-crosslinking and protein interactions	Chondrocytes	Cartilage	Li and Guan 2011
5	PVA	Chemical crosslinking	Chondrocytes	Cartilage	Yuan et al. 2017
6	PHEMA	Chemical crosslinking	Myoblasts	Skeletal muscles	Huang et al. 2013
7	PHEMA-MMA	Chemical crosslinkers	Chondrocytes	Cartilage	Tsai et al. 2006
8	PEO-Semi IPN	Chemical crosslinkers	Chondrocytes	Cartilage	Zoratto and Matricardi 2018
9	DEX-MA-AD	Chemical crosslinkers like aldehyde	ECs and SMCs	Vascular	Liu and Chan-Park 2009

and the resultant interpenetrating network was used for vascular tissue engineering [33]. A comparative study on hydrogels of fibrin/polyethylene oxide (PEO) serum albumin and the interpenetrating network of the same combination functionalized with methacrylate have shown more cell adhesion and migration in the interpenetrating network. Besides the interpenetrating and semi-interpenetrating, hydrogels are also being explored in hybrid hydrogels such as double network hydrogels, double network hydrogels with dual polymers, and guest-host hydrogels [34].

C) **Double network hydrogels:** The double network possesses both high water content and high mechanical strength and toughness. They are developed by combining two networks of opposite physical natures, i.e. the first component is highly crosslinked polyelectrolytes and the other component is sparsely crosslinked neutral polymers. The double network hydrogels possess hardness, strength, and toughness. These properties make them the scaffold of choice for many types of tissue regeneration [35, 36]. The double network hydrogels may not resist the high and frequent fractures as well as tensile stresses. A dual network approach may be helpful in increasing the suitability of a double network. Besides toughness, the dual network polymers can be made self-healing [37, 38]. To make the double network hydrogels excellent in mechanical strength and biocompatibility, the compatibilities of different materials are being exploited to achieve biocompatible, fracture/slicing resistant, and self-healing hydrogels also known as supramolecular hydrogels [39].

D) **Decellularized hydrogels**: Extracellular matrix is one of the best niches for cellular proliferation, migration, and signaling. These facts attracted many researchers to ECM to explore its applications in tissue engineering. ECM includes a mesh of biomolecules such as polysaccharides, glycosaminoglycans, laminins, collagens, and fibronectins [40]. ECM plays an important role in differentiation, migration, proliferation, and maturation of cells, along with providing them mechanical support [41].

8.4.3 METHODS OF HYDROGEL PREPARATION

Hydrogels can be prepared by crosslinking of different materials. The crosslinking of polymers can be obtained by various chemical and physical methods. Figure 8.2 shows different methods of crosslinking used for hydrogels development.

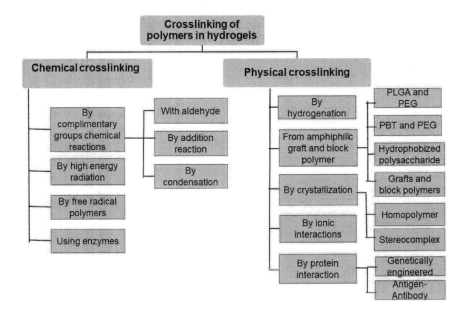

FIGURE 8.2   Types of crosslinking used for the preparation of hydrogels.

8.4.4 Properties of Hydrogels

An ideal hydrogel to be used in tissue engineering needs to possess several properties, including biocompatibility, biodegradability, porosity, and mechanical strength. A detailed discussion for each of these factors is provided in the following.

A) **Biocompatibility:** A definition for biocompatibility was accepted in the Chester Consensus Conference (1986) on Definitions in Biomaterials as "the ability of a material to perform with an appropriate host response in a specific application" [42]. Biocompatibility is essential as the transplants have problems of rejection. High doses of immunosuppressants are prescribed to the patients receiving transplants and may lead to further complications like immune-compromised patients [2, 43]. The materials used in tissue engineering can be processed to increase their biocompatibility and should be able to restore the tissue with expected functions, the phenotype of cells, and invisibility to immune response [43]. Scientists have tried to mimic the viruses and bacteria to escape the immune system and make them biocompatible for gene delivery applications [44]. The objective of studying biocompatibility of the material used in tissue engineering is that it should not have any toxic effect on the patient; there are three parameters that need to be considered in the evaluation of material: inflammation, immune response, and wound healing [43]. Implantation of scaffold or hydrogels triggers a foreign body reaction which leads to encapsulation of the implant by a fibrous capsule formed as a result of adhesion of various cells including monocytes, leukocytes, platelets, and non-specific protein adsorption on the surface of biomaterial or cytokine release [45].

B) **Biodegradability:** Hydrogels formulated for tissue engineering should be necessarily designed to be biodegradable so that complications of tissue scarring can be avoided or reduced [46]. The process of polymer degradation is attributed to the breakdown of bonds between monomers and polymers and usually occurs due to hydrolytic enzymes [47, 48]. The degradable monomers like poly (α-hydroxy acids) and poly (glycolic acid) make hydrogels too degradable [48, 49]. The addition of specific peptide sequences between macromers allows preparing hydrogels with enzyme cleavage sites. It can help in designing tissue-specific hydrogels that depend upon the presence of the enzyme in that tissue [21, 27]. The hydrogels were designed so that they can be hydrolyzed as well as enzymatically degraded upon addition of specific enzymes. This can help in maintaining the equilibrium in the rate of degradation of hydrogel with that of production of ECM by encapsulated cells [48, 50]. The degradation products also need to be considered while selecting the hydrogels as many materials have shown adverse effects on cells after degradation [51].

C) **Mechanical properties:** The mechanical behavior of hydrogels is typically viscoelastic, which is associated with the water and the movement of polymer networks in the fluid. It plays an important role in the behavior of cells, both at macroscopic and microscopic levels [48, 52]. Among other properties, the stiffness of a hydrogel is considered a key parameter that determines cell fate [53, 54]. In case of ECM, stiffness has shown the effect on human dermal fibroblasts growth, i.e. cells cultured on stiffer hydrogels proliferate faster and migrate slower compared to those cultured on soft substrates [55].

D) **Porosity of hydrogels:** Porosity plays a critical role in facilitating the transport of nutrients and oxygen for cell survival owing to the limited diffusion in hydrogels and along with the pore architecture and pore interconnectivity that play a crucial role in cell survival, proliferation, and migration [56, 57]. Another challenge encountered in the fabrication of hydrogel scaffolds is the inverse correlation between porosity and stiffness; an optimal balance is required to maintain the sufficient level of porosity to provide nutrients and oxygen while retaining the mechanical strength of the hydrogel [57]. Additionally, there is a direct correlation between the extent of secretion of the extracellular matrix and pore size [58]. The growth and penetration of cells in the 3D structure of the hydrogel are greatly affected by the average pore size of the hydrogel [56].

8.4.5. APPLICATION OF HYDROGELS IN TISSUE ENGINEERING

Hydrogels are considered valuable biomaterials for tissue engineering and tissue repair and have been studied extensively over the years for targeting various sites in the body. Neural tissue engineering is a fast-growing field which has the potential to alleviate problems associated with diseases, aging, or injury in the nervous system [59–61]. Figure 8.3 schematically shows the most common approaches currently being used clinically for tissue engineering applications. The general approach is to isolate the tissue-specific cells via a small biopsy from the patient and then expand them in vitro via cell culture, seeded into a well-designed scaffold and finally transplanted into the patient either through injection or via implantation at the desired site using surgery [62, 63].

Hyaluronic acid is present in the brain ECM, and hydrogels made up of hyaluronic acid and its modifications have shown better neural cell attachment [64]. In a study in rats, the hyaluronic acid scaffolds immobilized with arginine-glycine-aspartate (RGD) peptides supported cell infiltration, angiogenesis, and neurite extension and also showed minimization in glial scarring [65]. Hydrogels made up of collagen also have shown enhanced neural cell attachment as well as increase in cell viability. Although collagen does not naturally occur in the brain, it has been shown to support neural cell attachment and proliferation [25, 66–68].

Zhang et al. showed that 3D bioprinting using polymers like PCL and PLCL (50:50) with a spiral scaffold design demonstrated mechanical properties that were equivalent to the urethra in a rabbit and that cell-laden fibrin hydrogel led to active proliferation and maintained specific markers, thus providing a better microenvironment for cell growth and viability [69]. Young et al. demonstrated the feasibility of human lipoaspirate as an injectable adipose matrix scaffold for adipose tissue engineering, which was further extracted to generate a thermally responsive hydrogel. The results showed that human lipoaspirate was effectively decellularized and produced a self-assembling subcutaneous filler after

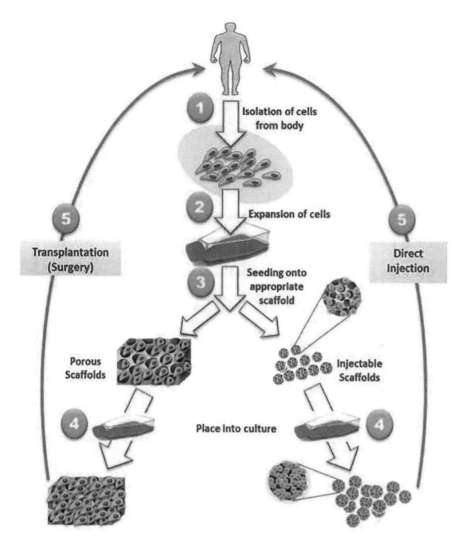

FIGURE 8.3   Schematic representation of tissue engineering approaches.

Source: [62].

subsequent solubilization [70]. The in situ polymerizing hydrogel-based adhesives have found their usage in repairing corneal injuries like perforations, the closing of the flap that arises due to LASIK surgery, and also successful corneal transplant [71]. If the biological imitating capacity of hydrogels with target tissue and cells is taken into consideration, it is highly possible to use hydrogels for successful ocular drug delivery. In fact, the biocompatible hydrogel can serve as a potential treatment for limbal stem cell deficiency (LSCD), where the ocular surface (OS) can be reconstructed by using autologous stem cells implanted in hydrogels [72].

Dunphy et al. performed a study which consisted of collagen-elastin constructs that were prepared with the goal of matching the properties of a single alveolar wall. The study showed how the addition of elastin affected the stiffness of collagen hydrogels, and the inclusion of lung fibroblasts in these constructs showed similar results to a single alveolar wall [73]. Also, Lee et al. investigated injectable collagen hydrogel for sustained ischemia/reperfusion injury and was able to facilitate recruitment of host stem cells into the kidney, which could contribute to the in situ regeneration of renal glomerular and tubular structures [74]. Manzoli et al. showed that both wild type and Green Fluorescent Protein (GFP)- human renal epithelial cells (hRECs) could be efficiently encapsulated within conformal hydrogel coatings through the fluid dynamic platform, which could be further refined by incorporating renal ECM as they showed improvement of cell viability and trophic factors secretion [75]. Loh et al. suggested novel thermosensitive hydrogel nanofiber scaffold mats fabricated by electrospinning, which showed temperature controlled release capabilities of the encapsulated drug or protein. Due to the resemblance to the extracellular matrix, these nanofiber mats proved to be excellent substrates for cell growth and adhesion along with more rapid hydrolytic degradation due to increased hydrophilicity [76]. A study explored the inclusion of both natural and synthetic biomaterials such as gelatin and methacrylate to form gelatin methacrylate (GelMA) photo-crosslinkable hydrogels for better resemblance to the extracellular matrix, which showed rapid cell adhesions and proteolytic degradability and their ability to enable surface binding and suggested that GelMA was well suited for creating vascularized engineered tissues [77].

A new class of bioactive scaffolds for tissue regeneration was prepared by Zhao et al. by forming in situ antibacterial and electroactive degradable hydrogels with quaternized chitosan grafted polyaniline with oxidized dextran as crosslinker, which showed good antibacterial activity for both gram-negative and gram-positive bacteria [78]. Miguel et al. developed a thermosensitive hydrogel consisting of chitosan/agarose, which showed improved healing with less scar formation and helped prevention of bacterial infection at the wound site that would make it suitable for use as a wound dressing [79]. Another study suggested the potential of novel injectable, biodegradable, self-healing hydrogels in repairing and healing the central nervous system deficits that included neurosphere-like progenitors, which could proliferate in the hydrogel and differentiate into neuron-like cells [80]. Mechanical strength is the most important factor in bone tissue engineering. The therapies involving regeneration of bones and cartilages are better treatments in degenerative diseases. Tissue engineering, where hydrogel scaffolds support the proliferation of chondrocytes and deliver the bioactive agent required for bone tissue regeneration, is a promising approach that can mimic the cartilage and bone ECM [81–83]. In the case of bone tissue engineering, composites of carbon nanotube and poly (lactic-co-glycolic acid) (PLGA) have shown promising results in various studies [84].

Natural hydrogels (e.g. hyaluronic acid and alginate) or synthetic polymers (e.g. PEG and methacrylate poly (glycerol succinic acid)) are being used for cartilage engineering. These hydrogels have supported the proliferation of chondrocytes as well as growth in cartilage tissue; the later ones showed better mechanical strength [85]. For successful tissue engineering, the mechanical strength in the scaffold is an essential factor in addition to morphology and viability of cells; thus, it should be one of the important criteria when selecting the scaffold material for hydrogel preparation in cartilage and bone tissue engineering.

Hydrogels are attractive materials for regeneration of the damaged myocardium as they provide mechanical support for cardiac cells to deposit extracellular matrix and form the newly synthesized tissue as they degrade [86]. Fujimoto et al. prepared a combination of poly(N-isopropyl acrylamide (PNIPAAm), a temperature-sensitive polymer, along with hydroxyethyl methacrylate poly (trimethylene carbonate) and acrylic acid (AAc)-based hydrogel in the cardiac injection application for delivery into the myocardium, which showed prevention of ventricular dilation and improved contractile function [87]. In another study, resilin-like polypeptides (RLPs) were used as potential material for cardiovascular tissue engineering along with PEG to form hybrid hydrogels which successfully encapsulated human aortic adventitial fibroblast cells [88]. Annabi et al. synthesized photo-crosslinked methacrylate tropoelastin (MeTro) hydrogels using recombinant human tropoelastin, which supported the synchronous beating of cardiomyocytes in response to electrical field stimulation and was amenable to the microfabrication of a variety of micrometer-sized well-defined geometries [89].

8.5 LIMITATIONS OF TISSUE ENGINEERING

A major limitation of hydrogels includes the lack of mechanical strength, which plays a key role in the tissue regeneration process and has limited porosity and insufficient interconnectivity. Other disadvantages of processing hydrogels are the difficulty of shaping them in predesigned geometries and the difficulty in manufacturing patient-specific implants due to limited control over the external geometry [90]. The scaffolds formed by the conventional or classical approaches lack long-range microarchitectural channels. Another limitation includes the high cost and various clinical issues faced with the effective scale-up of the hydrogel. Limited information is available on the impact of size on the biocompatibility of nanodevices and nanomaterials-based hydrogels [21]. Another challenge that is encountered includes optimizing cell viability, specifically with hydrogels, which have low mechanical strength [91].

8.6 CONCLUSION AND FUTURE PROSPECTS OF TISSUE ENGINEERING

Currently, various newer techniques and materials are being explored to overcome not only the scientific but also fundamental issues such as economic, social, and ethical concerns that are associated with tissue engineering. Injectable hydrogels are currently being explored, which would be beneficial by indirectly injecting the material into the defect site to support cell infiltration and growth of tissue. Another approach currently being explored includes attaching specific ligands to recreate the native tissue environment that would provide better attachment of the hydrogel to the site of application. Newer techniques and materials need to be developed to improve the properties of hydrogels including biocompatibility, porosity, and various mechanical properties. More recently, hybrid hydrogel systems have been designed which consist of at least two distinct classes of molecules or materials and provide better results compared to the conventional hydrogels. With these growing advancements, hydrogels can be fabricated to include multiple functions, programmable responses, and sensitivity to several stimuli [92].

8.7 ACKNOWLEDGMENTS

Dr. Rahul Dev Jayant would like to acknowledge the financial support from NIH Grant (R03DA044877–03), The Campbell Foundation (Florida, US) and Office of Science, basic science pilot funding, School of Pharmacy, Texas Tech University Health Sciences Center (TTUHSC), Texas, US.

REFERENCES

[1] F. Berthiaume, T.J. Maguire, M.L. Yarmush, Tissue engineering and regenerative medicine: History, progress, and challenges, *Annual Review of Chemical and Biomolecular Engineering*, 2 (2011) 403–430.
[2] R. Langer, J.P. Vacanti, Tissue engineering, *Science*, 260 (1993) 920–926.
[3] S. Naahidi, M. Jafari, M. Logan, Y. Wang, Y. Yuan, H. Bae, B. Dixon, P. Chen, Biocompatibility of hydrogel-based scaffolds for tissue engineering applications, *Biotechnology Advances*, 35 (2017) 530–544.
[4] H. Shin, S. Jo, A.G. Mikos, Biomimetic materials for tissue engineering, *Biomaterials*, 24 (2003) 4353–4364.
[5] J.L. Drury, D.J. Mooney, Hydrogels for tissue engineering: Scaffold design variables and applications, *Biomaterials*, 24 (2003) 4337–4351.
[6] S.J. Lee, J.J. Yoo, A. Atala, Biomaterials and tissue engineering, in: B.W. Kim (Ed.) *Clinical Regenerative Medicine in Urology*, Springer Singapore, Singapore, 2018, pp. 17–51.
[7] A. Khademhosseini, R.J.N.P. Langer, A decade of progress in tissue engineering, *Nature protocols*, 11 (2016): 1775.
[8] A. Vashist, A. Kaushik, A. Ghosal, R. Nikkhah-Moshaie, A. Vashist, R.D. Jayant, M. Nair, Journey of hydrogels to nanogels: A decade after, in: *Nanogels for Biomedical Applications*, Royal Society of Chemistry 2017, pp. 1–8.
[9] F.J. O'brien, Biomaterials & scaffolds for tissue engineering, *Materials Today*, 14 (2011) 88–95.
[10] U. Jammalamadaka, K. Tappa, Recent advances in biomaterials for 3D printing and tissue engineering, *Journal of Functional Biomaterials*, 9 (2018).
[11] D. Steffens, D.I. Braghirolli, N. Maurmann, P. Pranke, Update on the main use of biomaterials and techniques associated with tissue engineering, *Drug Discovery Today*, 23 (2018) 1474–1488.
[12] P.A. Gunatillake, R. Adhikari, Biodegradable synthetic polymers for tissue engineering, *European Cells and Materials*, 5 (2003) 1–16.
[13] N. Iqbal, A.S. Khan, A. Asif, M. Yar, J.W. Haycock, I.U. Rehman, Recent concepts in biodegradable polymers for tissue engineering paradigms: A critical review, *International Materials Reviews*, 64 (2019) 91–126.
[14] P. Zarrintaj, S. Manouchehri, Z. Ahmadi, M.R. Saeb, A.M. Urbanska, D.L. Kaplan, M. Mozafari, Agarose-based biomaterials for tissue engineering, *Carbohydrate Polymers*, 187 (2018) 66–84.
[15] A. Vedadghavami, F. Minooei, M.H. Mohammadi, S. Khetani, A. Rezaei Kolahchi, S. Mashayekhan, A. Sanati-Nezhad, Manufacturing of hydrogel biomaterials with controlled mechanical properties for tissue engineering applications, *Acta Biomaterialia*, 62 (2017) 42–63.

[16] E.J. Lee, F.K. Kasper, A.G. Mikos, Biomaterials for tissue engineering, *Annals of Biomedical Engineering*, 42 (2014) 323–337.

[17] B. Guo, P.X. Ma, Conducting polymers for tissue engineering, *Biomacromolecules*, 19 (2018) 1764–1782.

[18] P. Zarrintaj, B. Bakhshandeh, M.R. Saeb, F. Sefat, I. Rezaeian, M.R. Ganjali, S. Ramakrishna, M. Mozafari, Oligoaniline-based conductive biomaterials for tissue engineering, *Acta Biomaterialia*, 72 (2018) 16–34.

[19] A. Ghosal, A. Vashist, S. Tiwari, A. Kaushik, R.D. Jayant, M. Nair, J. Bhattacharya, Hydrogels: Smart nanomaterials for biomedical applications, in: *Synthesis of Inorganic Nanomaterials*, Elsevier, 2018, pp. 283–292.

[20] H.K. Ju, S.Y. Kim, S.J. Kim, Y.M. Lee, pH/temperature-responsive semi-IPN hydrogels composed of alginate and poly (N-isopropylacrylamide), *Journal of Applied Polymer Science*, 83 (2002) 1128–1139.

[21] J. Kopecek, Hydrogel biomaterials: A smart future? *Biomaterials*, 28 (2007) 5185–5192.

[22] M.P. Lutolf, Biomaterials: Spotlight on hydrogels, *Nature Materials*, 8 (2009) 451–453.

[23] J. Zhu, Bioactive modification of poly(ethylene glycol) hydrogels for tissue engineering, *Biomaterials*, 31 (2010) 4639–4656.

[24] F. Brandl, F. Sommer, A. Goepferich, Rational design of hydrogels for tissue engineering: Impact of physical factors on cell behavior, *Biomaterials*, 28 (2007) 134–146.

[25] J. Li, D.J. Mooney, Designing hydrogels for controlled drug delivery, *Nature Reviews Materials*, 1 (2016).

[26] V. Guarino, R. Altobelli, F. della Sala, A. Borzacchiello, L. Ambrosio, Alginate processing routes to fabricate bioinspired platforms for tissue engineering and drug delivery, in: *Alginates and Their Biomedical Applications*, Springer, New York, 2018, pp. 101–120.

[27] C.R. Nuttelman, M.A. Rice, A.E. Rydholm, C.N. Salinas, D.N. Shah, K.S. Anseth, Macromolecular monomers for the synthesis of hydrogel niches and their application in cell encapsulation and tissue engineering, *Progress in Polymer Science*, 33 (2008) 167–179.

[28] X. Jia, K.L. Kiick, Hybrid multicomponent hydrogels for tissue engineering, *Macromolecular Bioscience*, 9 (2009) 140–156.

[29] C. Hiemstra, L.J. Aa, Z. Zhong, P.J. Dijkstra, J. Feijen, Rapidly in situ-forming degradable hydrogels from dextran thiols through Michael addition, *Biomacromolecules*, 8 (2007) 1548–1556.

[30] R. Jin, L.S. Moreira Teixeira, A. Krouwels, P.J. Dijkstra, C.A. van Blitterswijk, M. Karperien, J. Feijen, Synthesis and characterization of hyaluronic acid-poly(ethylene glycol) hydrogels via Michael addition: An injectable biomaterial for cartilage repair, *Acta Biomaterialia*, 6 (2010) 1968–1977.

[31] J. Zhu, R.E. Marchant, Design properties of hydrogel tissue-engineering scaffolds, *Expert Review of Medical Devices*, 8 (2011) 607–626.

[32] P. Matricardi, C. Di Meo, T. Coviello, W.E. Hennink, F. Alhaique, Interpenetrating polymer networks polysaccharide hydrogels for drug delivery and tissue engineering, *Advanced Drug Delivery Reviews*, 65 (2013) 1172–1187.

[33] Y. Liu, M.B. Chan-Park, Hydrogel based on interpenetrating polymer networks of dextran and gelatin for vascular tissue engineering, *Biomaterials*, 30 (2009) 196–207.

[34] O. Gsib, J.L. Duval, M. Goczkowski, M. Deneufchatel, O. Fichet, V. Larreta-Garde, S.A. Bencherif, C. Egles, Evaluation of fibrin-based interpenetrating polymer networks as potential biomaterials for tissue engineering, *Nanomaterials* (Basel), 7 (2017).

[35] Q. Chen, H. Chen, L. Zhu, J. Zheng, Fundamentals of double network hydrogels, *Journal of Materials Chemistry B*, 3 (2015) 3654–3676.

[36] J.P. Gong, Why are double network hydrogels so tough? *Soft Matter*, 6 (2010) 2583–2590.

[37] N. Yuan, L. Xu, H. Wang, Y. Fu, Z. Zhang, L. Liu, C. Wang, J. Zhao, J. Rong, Dual physically cross-linked double network hydrogels with high mechanical strength, fatigue resistance, notch-insensitivity, and self-healing properties, *ACS Applied Materials & Interfaces*, 8 (2016) 34034–34044.

[38] X. Li, Q. Yang, Y. Zhao, S. Long, J. Zheng, Dual physically crosslinked double network hydrogels with high toughness and self-healing properties, *Soft Matter*, 13 (2017) 911–920.

[39] M. Fumagalli, K. Belal, H. Guo, F. Stoffelbach, G. Cooke, A. Marcellan, P. Woisel, D. Hourdet, Supramolecular polymer hydrogels induced by host—guest interactions with di-[cyclobis(paraquat-p-phenylene)] cross-linkers: From molecular complexation to viscoelastic properties, *Soft Matter*, 13 (2017) 5269–5282.

[40] A.D. Theocharis, S.S. Skandalis, C. Gialeli, N.K. Karamanos, Extracellular matrix structure, *Advanced Drug Delivery Reviews*, 97 (2016) 4–27.

[41] J. Labat-Robert, Cell-Matrix interactions, the role of fibronectin and integrins: A survey, *Pathologie Biologie* (Paris), 60 (2012) 15–19.

[42] R. Eloy, Challenges in biocompatibility and failure of biomaterials, in: *Biocompatibility and Performance of Medical Devices*, Elsevier, 2012, pp. 18–29.

[43] J.M. Anderson, Biocompatibility and bioresponse to biomaterials, in: *Principles of Regenerative Medicine*, Elsevier, 2019, pp. 675–694.

[44] M.T. Novak, J.D. Bryers, W.M. Reichert, Biomimetic strategies based on viruses and bacteria for the development of immune evasive biomaterials, *Biomaterials*, 30 (2009) 1989–2005.

[45] J.M. Anderson, A. Rodriguez, D.T. Chang, Foreign body reaction to biomaterials, *Seminars in Immunology*, 20 (2008) 86–100.

[46] D.J. Edell, V.V. Toi, V.M. McNeil, L.D. Clark, Factors influencing the biocompatibility of insertable silicon microshafts in cerebral cortex, *IEEE Transactions on Biomedical Engineering*, 39 (1992) 635–643.

[47] A. Metters, K. Anseth, C.J.P. Bowman, Fundamental studies of a novel, *Biodegradable PEG-b-PLA Hydrogel*, 41 (2000) 3993–4004.

[48] K.S. Anseth, A.T. Metters, S.J. Bryant, P.J. Martens, J.H. Elisseeff, C.N. Bowman, In situ forming degradable networks and their application in tissue engineering and drug delivery, *Journal of Controlled Release*, 78 (2002) 199–209.

[49] A.S. Sawhney, C.P. Pathak, J.A.J.M. Hubbell, Bioerodible hydrogels based on photopolymerized poly (ethylene glycol)-co-poly (. alpha.-hydroxy acid) diacrylate macromers, *Macromolecules*, 26 (1993) 581–587.

[50] M.A. Rice, J. Sanchez-Adams, K.S. Anseth, Exogenously triggered, enzymatic degradation of photopolymerized hydrogels with polycaprolactone subunits: Experimental observation and modeling of mass loss behavior, *Biomacromolecules*, 7 (2006) 1968–1975.

[51] E.L. Hedberg, H.C. Kroese-Deutman, C.K. Shih, R.S. Crowther, D.H. Carney, A.G. Mikos, J.A. Jansen, In vivo degradation of porous poly(propylene fumarate)/poly(DL-lactic-co-glycolic acid) composite scaffolds, *Biomaterials*, 26 (2005) 4616–4623.

[52] M.W. Tibbitt, K.S. Anseth, Hydrogels as extracellular matrix mimics for 3D cell culture, *Biotechnology and Bioengineering*, 103 (2009) 655–663.

[53] D.A. Rennerfeldt, A.N. Renth, Z. Talata, S.H. Gehrke, M.S. Detamore, Tuning mechanical performance of poly(ethylene glycol) and agarose interpenetrating network hydrogels for cartilage tissue engineering, *Biomaterials*, 34 (2013) 8241–8257.

[54] S. Nam, K.H. Hu, M.J. Butte, O. Chaudhuri, Strain-enhanced stress relaxation impacts nonlinear elasticity in collagen gels, *Proceedings of the National Academy of Sciences of the United States of America*, 113 (2016) 5492–5497.

[55] M.E. Smithmyer, L.A. Sawicki, A.M. Kloxin, Hydrogel scaffolds as in vitro models to study fibroblast activation in wound healing and disease, *Biomaterials Science*, 2 (2014) 634–650.

[56] N. Annabi, J.W. Nichol, X. Zhong, C. Ji, S. Koshy, A. Khademhosseini, F. Dehghani, Controlling the porosity and microarchitecture of hydrogels for tissue engineering, *Tissue Engineering: Part B, Reviews*, 16 (2010) 371–383.

[57] X. Guan, M. Avci-Adali, E. Alarcin, H. Cheng, S.S. Kashaf, Y. Li, A. Chawla, H.L. Jang, A. Khademhosseini, Development of hydrogels for regenerative engineering, *Biotechnology Journal*, 12 (2017).

[58] S.M. Lien, L.Y. Ko, T.J. Huang, Effect of pore size on ECM secretion and cell growth in gelatin scaffold for articular cartilage tissue engineering, *Acta Biomaterialia*, 5 (2009) 670–679.

[59] D.K. Cullen, J.A. Wolf, D.H. Smith, B.J. Pfister, Neural tissue engineering for neuroregeneration and biohybridized interface microsystems in vivo (Part 2), *Critical Reviews in Biomedical Engineering*, 39 (2011) 241–259.

[60] P. Sensharma, G. Madhumathi, R.D. Jayant, A.K.J.M.S. Jaiswal, E. C, Biomaterials and cells for neural tissue engineering: Current choices, *Materials Science and Engineering: C*, 77 (2017) 1302–1315.

[61] A. Vashist, A. Kaushik, A. Vashist, R.D. Jayant, A. Tomitaka, S. Ahmad, Y. Gupta, M.J.B.s. Nair, Recent trends on hydrogel based drug delivery systems for infectious diseases, *Biomaterials science*, 4 (2016) 1535–1553.

[62] I.M. El-Sherbiny, M.H.J.G.C.S. Yacoub, Practice, hydrogel scaffolds for tissue engineering: Progress and challenges, *Global Cardiology Science and Practice*, (2013) 38.

[63] A. Vashist, A. Kaushik, K. Alexis, R. Dev Jayant, V. Sagar, A. Vashist, M. Nair, Bioresponsive injectable hydrogels for on-demand drug release and tissue engineering, *Current pharmaceutical design*, 23 (2017) 3595–3602.

[64] L. Pan, Y. Ren, F. Cui, Q. Xu, Viability and differentiation of neural precursors on hyaluronic acid hydrogel scaffold, *Journal of Neuroscience Research*, 87 (2009) 3207–3220.

[65] F.Z. Cui, W.M. Tian, S.P. Hou, Q.Y. Xu, I.S. Lee, Hyaluronic acid hydrogel immobilized with RGD peptides for brain tissue engineering, *Journal of Materials Science: Materials in Medicine*, 17 (2006) 1393–1401.

[66] K.E. Kadler, C. Baldock, J. Bella, R.P. Boot-Handford, Collagens at a glance, *Journal of cell science*, 120 (2007) 1955–1958.

[67] M.J. Mahoney, C. Krewson, J. Miller, W.M. Saltzman, Impact of cell type and density on nerve growth factor distribution and bioactivity in 3-dimensional collagen gel cultures, *Tissue Engineering*, 12 (2006) 1915–1927.

[68] S.H. Bhang, T.J. Lee, J.M. Lim, J.S. Lim, A.M. Han, C.Y. Choi, Y.H. Kwon, B.S. Kim, The effect of the controlled release of nerve growth factor from collagen gel on the efficiency of neural cell culture, *Biomaterials*, 30 (2009) 126–132.

[69] K. Zhang, Q. Fu, J. Yoo, X. Chen, P. Chandra, X. Mo, L. Song, A. Atala, W. Zhao, 3D bioprinting of urethra with PCL/PLCL blend and dual autologous cells in fibrin hydrogel: An in vitro evaluation of biomimetic mechanical property and cell growth environment, *Acta Biomaterialia*, 50 (2017) 154–164.

[70] D.A. Young, D.O. Ibrahim, D. Hu, K.L. Christman, Injectable hydrogel scaffold from decellularized human lipoaspirate, *Acta Biomaterialia*, 7 (2011) 1040–1049.

[71] M.W. Grinstaff, Designing hydrogel adhesives for corneal wound repair, *Biomaterials*, 28 (2007) 5205–5214.

[72] M. Fathi, J. Barar, A. Aghanejad, Y. Omidi, Hydrogels for ocular drug delivery and tissue engineering, *Bioimpacts*, 5 (2015) 159–164.

[73] S.E. Dunphy, J.A. Bratt, K.M. Akram, N.R. Forsyth, A.J. El Haj, Hydrogels for lung tissue engineering: Biomechanical properties of thin collagen-elastin constructs, *Journal of the Mechanical Behavior of Biomedical Materials*, 38 (2014) 251–259.

[74] S.J. Lee, H.J. Wang, T.H. Kim, J.S. Choi, G. Kulkarni, J.D. Jackson, A. Atala, J.J. Yoo, In situ tissue regeneration of renal tissue induced by collagen hydrogel injection, *Stem Cells Translational Medicine*, 7 (2018) 241–250.

[75] V. Manzoli, D.C. Colter, S. Dhanaraj, A. Fornoni, C. Ricordi, A. Pileggi, A.A. Tomei, Engineering human renal epithelial cells for transplantation in regenerative medicine, *Medical Engineering & Physics*, 48 (2017) 3–13.

[76] X.J. Loh, P. Peh, S. Liao, C. Sng, J. Li, Controlled drug release from biodegradable thermoresponsive physical hydrogel nanofibers, *Journal of Controlled Release*, 143 (2010) 175–182.

[77] J.W. Nichol, S.T. Koshy, H. Bae, C.M. Hwang, S. Yamanlar, A. Khademhosseini, Cell-laden microengineered gelatin methacrylate hydrogels, *Biomaterials*, 31 (2010) 5536–5544.

[78] X. Zhao, P. Li, B. Guo, P.X. Ma, Antibacterial and conductive injectable hydrogels based on quaternized chitosan-graft-polyaniline/oxidized dextran for tissue engineering, *Acta Biomaterialia*, 26 (2015) 236–248.

[79] T.C. Tseng, L. Tao, F.Y. Hsieh, Y. Wei, I.M. Chiu, S.H. Hsu, An injectable, self-healing hydrogel to repair the central nervous system, *Advanced Materials*, 27 (2015) 3518–3524.

[80] S.P. Miguel, M.P. Ribeiro, H. Brancal, P. Coutinho, I.J. Correia, Thermoresponsive chitosan-agarose hydrogel for skin regeneration, *Carbohydrate Polymers*, 111 (2014) 366–373.

[81] E. Alsberg, K.W. Anderson, A. Albeiruti, R.T. Franceschi, D.J. Mooney, Cell-interactive alginate hydrogels for bone tissue engineering, *Journal of Dental Research*, 80 (2001) 2025–2029.

[82] J.M. Mason, A.S. Breitbart, M. Barcia, D. Porti, R.G. Pergolizzi, D.A. Grande, Cartilage and bone regeneration using gene-enhanced tissue engineering, *Clinical Orthopaedics and Related Research*, (2000) S171–178.

[83] J.A. Burdick, K.S. Anseth, Photoencapsulation of osteoblasts in injectable RGD-modified PEG hydrogels for bone tissue engineering, *Biomaterials*, 23 (2002) 4315–4323.

[84] P.E. Mikael, A.R. Amini, J. Basu, M. Josefina Arellano-Jimenez, C.T. Laurencin, M.M. Sanders, C. Barry Carter, S.P. Nukavarapu, Functionalized carbon nanotube reinforced scaffolds for bone regenerative engineering: Fabrication, in vitro and in vivo evaluation, *Biomedical Materials*, 9 (2014) 035001.

[85] M. Yamamoto, Y. Ikada, Y. Tabata, Controlled release of growth factors based on biodegradation of gelatin hydrogel, *Journal of Biomaterials Science, Polymer Edition*, 12 (2001) 77–88.

[86] G. Camci-Unal, N. Annabi, M.R. Dokmeci, R. Liao, A. Khademhosseini, Hydrogels for cardiac tissue engineering, *NPG Asia Materials*, 6 (2014) e99.

[87] K.L. Fujimoto, Z. Ma, D.M. Nelson, R. Hashizume, J. Guan, K. Tobita, W.R. Wagner, Synthesis, characterization and therapeutic efficacy of a biodegradable, thermoresponsive hydrogel designed for application in chronic infarcted myocardium, *Biomaterials*, 30 (2009) 4357–4368.

[88] C.L. McGann, E.A. Levenson, K.L. Kiick, Resilin-based hybrid hydrogels for cardiovascular tissue engineering, *Macromolecules*, 214 (2013) 203–213.

[89] N. Annabi, K. Tsang, S.M. Mithieux, M. Nikkhah, A. Ameri, A. Khademhosseini, A.S. Weiss, Highly elastic micropatterned hydrogel for engineering functional cardiac tissue, *Advanced Functional Materials*, 23 (2013).

[90] T. Billiet, M. Vandenhaute, J. Schelfhout, S. Van Vlierberghe, P. Dubruel, A review of trends and limitations in hydrogel-rapid prototyping for tissue engineering, *Biomaterials*, 33 (2012) 6020–6041.

[91] O. Tao, D.T. Wu, H.M. Pham, N. Pandey, S.D.J.A.S. Tran, Nanomaterials in craniofacial tissue regeneration: A review, *Applied Sciences*, 9 (2019) 317.

[92] N. Saha, N. Saha, T. Sáha, P. Sáha, Importance of multi-stakeholder initiatives in applications of bacterial cellulose-based hydrogels for sustainable development In: Mondal M. (eds) Cellulose-Based Superabsorbent Hydrogels. Polymers and Polymeric Composites: A Reference Series. Springer, *Cham*, (2019) 1277–1301 5.

9 Antibacterial Hydrogels and Their Implications

Jyoti Bala, Anupam J. Das, and Ajeet Kaushik

CONTENTS

9.1 INTRODUCTION

Antimicrobial resistance (AMR) is the ability of microorganisms to resist the effects of a drug that were previously effectively treating the microbe [1–3]. Antibiotics have been extensively used in the antibacterial field and have significantly improved the quality of life for human beings by effectively suppressing various infections [4–6]. Antibiotic resistance happens when bacteria develop resistance against antibiotics, which thereby reduces or eliminates the effectiveness of antibacterial drugs. The bacteria survive and continue to multiply, causing more harm and making prevention and treatment a tedious task, hence making AMR a challenging global issue [7–10]. Antibiotics are well known for their crucial roles and applications. But their wrong use causes abuse and leads to major health concerns. The overuse and misuse of antibiotics and the reduced amount of novel antimicrobial drug development are a major cause of the aggravation of this crisis. Microbial resistance to multiple drugs is known as multidrug-resistant (MDR) whereas extensively drug-resistant (XDR) is often termed "superbugs" [11–14]. Conventional antibacterial treatments are ineffective, and infections persist due to antibiotic resistance. The instant emergence of antibiotic-resistant bacteria almost after the advanced antibiotics approval was challenging in cases of Fidaxomicin-resistant *Enterococci* (K-1476) and Methicillin-resistant *Staphylococcus aureus* (MRSA) [15]. Pathogens like *Pseudomonas aeruginosa*, *Staphylococcus aureus*, and *Escherichia coli* pose severe health concerns. Wound healing delay, sepsis of the affected site, occurrence of pneumonia, complications for ICU patients, transplant rejection, or even severe internal infections which are hard to detect and difficult to treat can be caused by AMR [16–20]. Global threats from AMR pathogenic microorganisms trigger the need for the advancement and development of novel antibacterial materials. In this context, recently several biomaterials and hydrogels have been synthesized, investigated, and characterized for their effective and efficient antibacterial activities. Hydrogels are smart materials which can represent antibacterial activities and can act as novel agents in the fight against AMR [21–24]. Hydrogel contains very high amounts of water and a specific structural complexity. Hydrogels are cross-linked polymer networks formed by either physical interactions or covalent bonds according to the change in diverse parameters such as pH, ionic strength, ultraviolet exposure, temperature, etc. [25–27]. Hydrogel has broad applications in diverse fields such as wound healing/dressing, three-dimensional (3D) cell culture systems, tissue engineering, bioengineering, nanomedicine, and drug delivery [28–33]. Their better biocompatibility, higher adsorbent quality, and the feasibility to design and modify the hydrogels to mimic extracellular structures or specific parts of tissues makes them potential candidates for biomedical applications. Several nanomaterials based on metal ions and other bionanomaterials were discovered and investigated for their antibacterial activity [34–38]. In this chapter, we have reviewed the different types of antibacterial hydrogels and their implications, applications, and potential future scope.

9.2 HYDROGELS AS ANTIBACTERIAL AGENT AND THEIR IMPLICATIONS

Hydrogels are natural or synthetic porous materials which consist of cross-linked polymers formed by either physical or chemical interaction [22, 23, 39]. Recently hydrogels have been comprehensively considered and implemented as an alternative material for antibacterial applications [29, 40–42]. There are mainly three classes of antibacterial hydrogels (Figure 9.1). These are inorganic nanoparticle-containing hydrogels (metal or metal oxide), antibacterial (antibiotics)-containing hydrogels, and inherent hydrogel (natural or synthetic) with antibacterial capabilities. The properties of hydrogels, such as hydrophilicity and porosity, have been utilized for

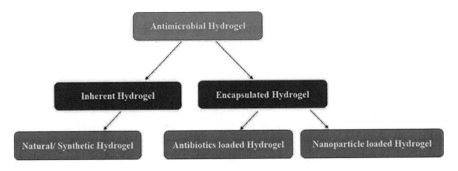

FIGURE 9.1 Schematic overview of various types of antimicrobial hydrogels.

the development of effective antibacterial candidates and drug delivery purposes. Antibacterial hydrogels could help resolve the challenges of antibiotic resistance. Antibacterial hydrogels could be used locally to avoid the side effects of systemic application. Antibacterial hydrogels, as a novel drug delivery system, offer sustainable release and prolonged antibacterial consequence. Additionally, synergestic application has advantages over aiming at a single target. However, multiple mechanisms involved with nanoparticles and other antibacterial constituents intricates the development of bacterial resistance. Thus, making hydrogels as a smart alternative to fight AMR varied component might exhibit synergistic effects which could provide broader antibacterial spectrum and effective antibacterial activity. High selectivity and negligible toxicity of these hydrogels would make them great impending candidates in the prevention and treatment of infections [43–45].

9.3 APPLICATION OF ANTIBACTERIAL HYDROGELS

Applications and implication of several antibacterial hydrogel formulations are provided in this section. Briefly, antibacterial hydrogels can be divided into three groups. Hydrogels as antibacterial agent can acquiescently substitute conventional antibiotic treatments. Antibacterial hydrogels can be widely applied in the field of wound healing, urinary tract infection, gastrointestinal infections, osteomyelitis, skin infection, catheter-associated infections, and contact lenses [32, 46–50].

9.3.1 Inorganic Nanoparticle-Containing Hydrogels

Inorganic antibacterial agents primarily include frequently used metal ions and metal oxide nanoparticles such as gold (Au), copper (Cu), silver (Ag), zinc oxide (ZnO), and nickel oxide (NiO) [51–54]. Hydrogels incorporating inorganic antibacterial material enhance the antibacterial properties for prolonged period, making them an efficient antibacterial agent. The mode of action of antibacterial metal and metallic nanoparticles is speculative and is believed to be due to their ability to damage the bacterial cell membrane and affect other bacterial organelles. Ag has long been known for its antimicrobial activity and its application in biomedical sectors such as wound healing, bone implants, bacterial infection treatment, etc. With the advancement of nanotechnology, Ag-based nanoparticles and bionanomaterial have been synthesized and characterized for various properties including its antibacterial, anticancer, and antimicrobial activities. The antibacterial property of Ag is well established although the mechanisms of its action still remain uncertain. It is hypothesized that the Ag ion (Ag^+) can bind to the bacterial cell membrane by Ag^+ and the thiol group interaction, consequently affecting the bacterial cell's viability and subsequently inhibiting the replication of DNA. Polysaccharide-based natural hydrogels incorporated Ag Nanoparticles (NPs) were reported by Stojkovska et al., such alginate based natural polysaccharides are widely used for the synthesis of hydrogels via ionic interactions with Ca^{2+}. They have synthesized Ag NPs sodium alginate microbeads based hydrogel using electrochemical method which were used against the *S. aureus bacteria*. Chu and Hang (2019) have undertaken injectable hydrogel studies. Osteoinductive and osteoconductive superparamagnetic Fe_3O_4 nanoparticles (MNP) and hydroxyapatite (HAP) nanoparticles incorporated into a di-block copolymer-based thermo-responsive hydrogel, methoxy (polyethylene glycol)-polyalanine (mPA), were investigated. Functional characterization of integrated inorganic nanoparticles modulated biomarkers of bone differentiation and enhanced bone mineralization were shown. Their results exhibit the significance of using a combination of external (magnet) and internal (scaffold) magnetism for bone regeneration. Furthermore, Madhusudana Rao et al. demonstrated sodium alginate (SA)-based semi-interpenetrating polymer network hydrogels for the incorporation of Ag NPs. Their results establish the antibacterial role of Ag nanocomposite hydrogels which could be used for biomedical and clinical relevance. In another study, Pasqi et al. showed the synthesis of composite hydrogels containing carboxymethyl cellulose (CMC) polymer chains and TiO_2 NPs functionalized with amine groups. These NPs served as cross-linkers in the hydrogel and thus contributed mechanical amends to the hybrid gels and proposed its scope in medical and tissue engineering [55]. Gelatin/Ag, pectin/hydroxyethyl methacrylate/TiO_2, and chitosan/Au hydrogel composites have also been reported by others [56]. Additionally, Neibert et al. described a strategy to augment the mechanical strength of SA hydrogel loaded with Ag NPs. Briefly, calcium- or N,N-methylenebisacrylamide-cross-linked SA fibers were incorporated with Ag NPs, which was investigated for its biological role in wound dressings or healing application [57].

9.3.2 ANTIBIOTIC-CONTAINING HYDROGELS

Alvarez et al. have suggested that antibiotic-loaded silica NP-collagen composite hydrogels provide prolonged antimicrobial activity for wound infection prevention [58]. Briefly, Gentamicin and Rifamycin were encapsulated in a single step within plain silica nanoparticles, and their biological roles were characterized against *Pseudomonas aeruginosa* and *Staphylococcus aureus*. Gentamicin prolonged release from the nanocomposites sustained over 7 days and thereby resulted in tremendous antibacterial activity and also with lesser cytotoxicity towards surface-seeded fibroblast cells. They have concluded that the complex interplay of interactions among drugs, silica, and collagen is a crucial factor regulating the properties and activity of these composite hydrogels. Ciprofloxacin (CIP) is a fluoroquinolone-based antibiotic with a broad antibacterial spectrum against both gram-positive and gram-negative bacteria [59]. CIP antibacterial property is considered due to its ability to block DNA duplication by binding the DNA gyrases and causing a double-stranded break in bacterial chromosome. CIP-loaded hydrogel has been developed and has prospects in prevention of several infections. CIP assembled with a tripeptide (d-Leu-Phe-Phe) and incorporated into hydrogels has high drug loading efficiency (DLE), which provides efficient prolonged release. Moreover, CIP-peptide self-assembled hydrogel demonstrated high antimicrobial activity against *S. aureus*, *E. coli*, and *Klebsiella pneumonia* with no cytotoxicity during hemolysis assays of red blood cells or in cultures of fibroblast cells. In another study, hydrogel synthesized by the polymerization of 3-aminophenylboronic acid with PVA for CIP incorporation has demonstrated antimicrobial activity and wound healing in diabetes patients [60].

Shukla and Shukla (2018) have shown tunable antibiotic delivery from gellan hydrogels. They have synthesized two types of hydrogels using 1% w/v gellan and 1 mM $CaCl_2$ "ointment" hydrogels and those formed by using 4% w/v gellan and 7 mM $CaCl_2$ "sheet" hydrogels [61].Vancomycin, another broad-spectrum antibiotic, was incorporated in hydrogels via direct and/or as in graphitized carbon black nanoparticles (CNPs). Prolonged release of sheet and ointment hydrogels was studied at suitable concentrations. Their data suggest that final drug release amounts are influenced by intermolecular interactions between Vancomycin and gellan. They have shown in vitro growth inhibition of *Staphylococcus aureus* and Methicillin-resistant *Staphylococcus aureus* in the presence of chosen hydrogels [62]. Remarkably, they have also found that these hydrogels are non-toxic to wound healing cells including fibroblasts and mesenchymal stem cells. Vancomycin (VAN) is considered the last form of defense against infection. The discovery of VAN-resistant *Enterococcus* is a crucial concern. Hydrogel has been investigated to tackle this challenge and control Vancomycin delivery. Gustafson et al. synthesized a charged hydrogel as a carrier that was incorporated with Vancomycin [63]. Additionally, various other antibiotic-loaded hydrogels have also been reported in past years such as (i) Ampicillin sodium-loaded PVA-SA hydrogel (gram-positive and gram-negative bacteria), and (ii) Cephalosporin antibiotic and Levo oxacin-loaded hyaluronic acid hydrogels for antibacterial activity [64–66]. Furthermore, Doxycycline (DOX)-loaded thermosensitive hydroxypropyl-β-cyclodextrin (HP-β-CD) hydrogels were also synthesized and characterized for ophthalmic delivery [67].

9.3.3 HYDROGELS WITH INHERENT ANTIBACTERIAL PROPERTIES

Hydrogels with inherent antibacterial properties are effective candidates containing antibacterial components [23, 32]. Several studies have been conducted in past years aiming to develop effective, cheap, and non-toxic inherent antibacterial hydrogels as discussed in the following section. Inherent hydrogels are of two types: natural and synthetic. Hydrogels with antibacterial polymer, antibacterial peptides, and amphoteric hydrogels are such examples. Kumar et al. have shown highly bactericidal macroporous polymeric hydrogel for water disinfection could also be applicable in other bacteria inactivation applications. Briefly, they have demonstrated an effective point-of-use (on-demand) water disinfection technology in the form of a polymeric scaffold called a macroporous antimicrobial polymeric gel (MAPG), which is easy to modify and less toxic with an inherent antimicrobial property. They have found that MAPG is an effective bactericidal and can disinfect bacteria-contaminated water (ca. 10^8 CFU mL^{-1}) at higher capacity, inactivating >99% of broad spectrum of bacteria including *Escherichia coli*, *Vibrio cholerae*, and *Staphylococcus aureus* [68]. Wu et al. 2018 have shown antibacterial coordinated polymer hydrogels composed of Ag-PEGylatedbisimidazolylbenzyl alcohol. These hydrogels exhibit higher antibacterial activity than silver nitrate against broad-spectrum pathogens and certain multidrug-resistant pathogens such as *Staphylococcus aureus* and methicillin-resistant *Staphylococcus aureus* [69]. Antibacterial polymers are often also categorized as non-stimulated antibacterial polymers and potential antibacterial polymers. Commonly non-stimulated antibacterial polymers contain structures that are significant for antibacterial activity. The polymer hydrogel contains thermo-responsive PNIPAM and redox-responsive polyferrocenylsilane macromolecules which are responsible for proficient antibacterial properties and additionally provide high biocompatibilities. Recently, redox-induced formation of hydrogel-Ag composites has suggested an antimicrobial role of these hydrogels against *E. coli*. Recently, P(HEMA/IA), pH-sensitive and thermal-sensitive hydrogels could inhibit the entry of *S. aureus* and *E. coli*, with potential scope in the biomedical sector such as in skin treatment and wound healing [70]. Interestingly, no evidence of cell toxicity or considerable hemolytic activity was observed during in vitro study of P(HEMA/IA) biocompatibility. Peptide-based hydrogels are natural antibacterial hydrogels that have gained consideration after the discovery of antimicrobial peptides (AMPs). They are generally amphiphilic and possess a cationic charge, enabling electrostatic interactions with anionic bacterial membranes and subsequently leading to membrane disruption and bacterial death [72–74]. Although AMPs cannot self-assemble into a hydrogel, novel peptides resembling the properties of AMPs are in development and can self-assemble into hydrogels under suitable conditions with desirable antimicrobial properties.

9.4 SUMMARY

Antibiotic resistance developed due to the exploitation of antibiotic drugs and is a global threat. Natural and synthetic hydrogels have either inherent antibacterial properties or execute as carriers for antibiotics. Hydrogels as antibacterial biomaterials are an unconventional and efficient agent that suppresses many drug-resistant bacteria [32–39]. Local control and prolonged release, local administration, specific on-off release, stability, and better biocompatibility are imperative which make hydrogels a smart choice as antibacterial candidates. It is crucial that antibacterial components can easily release from the gel and enter immune cells and subsequently inhibit the bacterial infection. Hydrogels loaded with antibiotics and antimicrobial polymers release the antimicrobial agents in a sustained way, enhancing the proficiently of treatment and preventing biofilm formation [75]. Biodegradable antibacterial polymer-loaded or peptide-loaded gels have an extra advantage over gels encapsulated with antibiotics or metal nanoparticles. Some of the hydrogels were investigated with specific bacteria while other hydrogels were considered with broad-spectrum gram-positive (*S. aureus*) and gram-negative bacteria (*E. coli*). The results suggested that the antimicrobial properties of hydrogels were different against diverse bacteria. Rarely, the entire antimicrobial spectrum of antibacterial hydrogels has been reported. Further studies about the antibacterial properties of antibacterial hydrogels against various bacteria will help researchers determine if their activity is against a broad spectrum and of wide utility. Interesting advancement has been done in this area; Nguyen et al. have demonstrated antibacterial chitosan/polyvinyl alcohol loaded with Ag nanoparticles hydrogel for wound healing [76]. Photodynamic PHEMA-based hydrogel, which can be light induced, has antibacterial activity through release of nitric oxide. These polymers have antibacterial properties but could also be used for responsive delivery and release methods [77]. Injectable gellan gum-based PLGA NP-loaded systems, injectable Pluronic-α-CD supramolecular gels (CD, cyclodextrin), and hydrogels consisting of thiolated chitosan cross-linked with maleic acid–grafted dextran are a few of the advanced antibacterial hydrogels [78–80]. Other smart hydrogels such as photo-cross-linked methacrylated dextran and poly(l-glutamic acid)-*graft*-hydroxyethyl methacrylate (PGA-*g*-HEMA) hydrogels were also reported, and both exhibited greater antibacterial properties and desirable release capabilities [81–84]. Other research focused on the hydrogels composed of polysaccharides, PEG, or other hydrophilic polymers in combination with different antibacterial substances [85–90]. For hydrogels to be utilized therapeutically, biocompatibility and biodegradability are crucial necessities. Furthermore, several hydrogels were also studied as drug carriers, for which hydrogels should have high DLE, lesser side effects, negligible toxicity, and no inflammation in biological samples. It is quite evident that smart hydrogels should be explored and utilized further to overcome the AMR challenge (Figure 9.2). Few challenges need to be focused on, such as inorganic antibacterial hydrogel agents like Ag NPs, which have good antibacterial properties but the inadequate biocompatibility and dosage dependency curtail their applications. Drug-resistant bacteria have evolved because of antibiotic abuse and other antibacterial drugs mishandling. Antibacterial hydrogels definitely provide a solution to the issue of bacterial resistance.

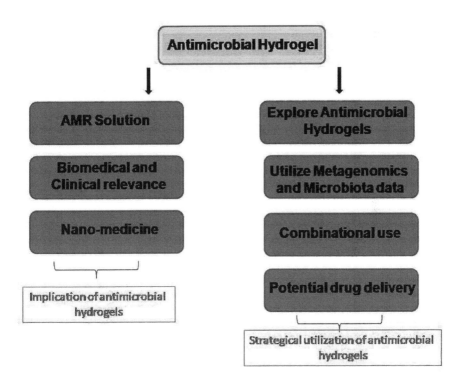

FIGURE 9.2 Schematic overview of implication of antimicrobial hydrogels and strategic utilization of smart antimicrobial hydrogels.

9.5   FUTURE PROSPECTS

Furthermore, antibacterial hydrogels have tremendous prospects in applied biomedical and clinical research. The use of novel antibacterial biomaterials and the combination of such materials could bring prospects promising scope for solving the AMR challenge. Further development of advanced effective antibacterial hydrogels could be of notable importance to fight the AMR challenge. Hydrogels have presented an exciting approach to scrap antibiotic resistance, though a few issues need to be addressed to provide accuracy in controlled release of drugs in the existing hydrogels. Some of the hydrogels degrade very rapidly, thus leading to prolong the effect. Additionally, the antibacterial property of hydrogels is usually less efficient and weak, thus preventing their convenient application. In the future, these problems should be addressed by further research. For future clinical applications, it is critical to investigate antimicrobial hydrogels against clinically isolated multidrug-resistant strains. With rational design, utilizing metagenomics data, microbiota data, synthetic polymer chemistry, and comprehensive evaluation studies, hydrogel and encapsulated cargos with broad-spectrum antimicrobial-resistant microbes could be tackled efficiently.

9.6   CONFLICT OF INTEREST

The authors declare no conflict of interest.

REFERENCES

[1]   Geneva: 1996. World Health Organization. The world health report (https://www.who.int/whr/1996/en/).
[2]   Raghunath D. Emerging antibiotic resistance in bacteria with special reference to India. *Journal of Biosciences*, 2008;33:593–603.
[3]   Davies J, Davies D. Origins and evolution of antibiotic resistance. *Microbiology and Molecular Biology Reviews* 2010;74:417–433.
[4]   Bush K. Antibacterial drug discovery in the 21st century. *Clinical Microbiology and Infection* 2004;10:10–17.
[5]   Amábile-Cuevas CF. New antibiotics and new resistance. *American Scientist* 2003; 91:138–149.
[6]   Aminov RI. The role of antibiotics and antibiotic resistance in nature. *Environmental Microbiology* 2009;11:2970–2988.
[7]   Adam M, Murali B, Glenn NO, Potter SS. Epigenetic inheritance based evolution of antibiotic resistance in bacteria. *BMC Evolutionary Biology* 2008;8:52. Doi:10.1186/1471-2148-8-52.
[8]   Calabrese EJ. Getting the dose—response wrong: why hormesis became marginalized and the threshold model accepted. *Archives of Toxicology*, 2009;83:227–247.
[9]   Zhu Y, Johnson TA., Su J, et al. Diverse and abundant antibiotic resistance genes in Chinese swine farms. *Proceedings of the National Academy of Sciences of the United States of America* 2013;110:3435–3440.
[10] Vargiu AV., Pos KM., Poole K, et al. Editorial: bad bugs in the XXIst century: resistance mediated by multi-drug efflux pumps in Gram-negative bacteria. *Frontiers in Microbiology* 2016;7:833.
[11] Ventola L. The antibiotic resistant crisis. *P&T.* 2015;40(4):277–283.

[12] Harbottle HS, Thakur S, Zhao S, White DG. Genetics of antimicrobial resistance. *Animal Biotechnology* 2006Pl;17:111–124.

[13] Parveen RM, Acharya NS, Dhodapkar R, Harish BN, Parija SC. Molecular epidemiology of Multidrug resistant Extended-Spectrum β-Lactamase Producing Klebsiellapneumoniae outbreak in a neonatal intensive care unit. *International Journal of Collaborative Research on Internal Medicine & Public Health* 2010;2:226–233.

[14] Bryskier A. *Antimicrobial Agents: Antibacterials and Antifungals.* Washington, DC: *American Society for Microbiology,* 2005.

[15] Tsering DC, Pal R, Kar S. Methicillin-resistant *Staphylococcus aureus*: prevalence and current susceptibility pattern in Sikkim. *Journal of global infectious diseases* 2011;3:9–13.

[16] Thind P, Prakash SK, Wadhwa A, Garg VK, Pati B. Bacteriological profile of community acquired pyoderma with special reference to methicillin resistant *Staphylococcus aureus. Indian Journal of Dermatology, Venereology and Leprology* 2010;76:572–574.

[17] Waness A. Revisiting methicillin-resistant *Staphylococcus aureus* infections. *Journal of global infectious diseases* 2010;2:49–56.

[18] Bhatia R, Narain JP. The growing challenge of antimicrobial resistance in the South-East Asia Region-Are we losing the battle? *Indian Journal of Medical Research* 2010;132:482–486.

[19] Jain A, Mandal R. Prevalence of antimicrobial resistance pattern of extended spectrum beta-lactamase producing Klebsiella species isolated from cases of neonatal septicemia. *Indian Journal of Medical Research* 2007;125:89–94.

[20] Loomba PS, Taneja J, Mishra B. Methicillin and vancomycin resistant *s. aureus* in hospitalized patients. *Journal of global infectious diseases* 2010;2:275–283.

[21] Ng VW, Chan JM, Sardon H, et al. Antimicrobial hydrogels: a new weapon in the arsenal against multidrug-resistant infections. *Advanced Drug Delivery Reviews* 2014;78:46–62.

[22] Malmsten M. Antimicrobial and antiviral hydrogels. *Soft Matter* 2011;7(19):8725.

[23] Dasgupta A, Mondal JH, Das D. Peptide hydrogels. *RSC Advances* 2013;3(24):9117.

[24] Pelgrift RY, Friedman AJ. Nanotechnology as a therapeutic tool to combat microbial resistance. *Advanced Drug Delivery Reviews* 2013;65(13–14):1803–1815.

[25] Wichterle O, Lím D. Hydrophilic gels for biological use. *Nature.* 1960;185:117–118.

[26] Haraguchi K, Takehisa T. Nanocomposite hydrogels: a unique organic-inorganic network structure with extraordinary mechanical, optical, and swelling/de-swelling properties. *Advanced Materials* 2002;14:1120–1124.

[27] Gong JP, Katsuyama Y, Kurokawa T, Osada Y. Double-network hydrogels with extremely high mechanical strength. *Advanced Materials* 2003;15:1155–1158.

[28] Haraguchi K, Li HJ, Okumura N. Hydrogels with hydrophobic surfaces: abnormally high contact angles for water on PNIPA nanocomposite hydrogels. *Macromolecules.* 2007;40:2299–2302.

[29] Chen J, Park H, Park K. Synthesis of superporous hydrogels: hydrogels with fast swelling and superabsorbent properties. *Journal of Biomedical Materials Research* 1999;44:53–62.

[30] Petka WA, Harden JL, McGrath KP, Wirtz D, Tirrell DA. Reversible hydrogels from self-assembling artificial proteins. *Science.* 1998;281:389–392.

[31] Xu C, Breedveld V, Kopeček J. Reversible hydrogels from self-assembling genetically engineered block copolymers. *Biomacromolecules.* 2005;6:1739–1749.

[32] García-Barrasa J, López-de-Luzuriaga JM, Monge M. Silver nanoparticles: synthesis through chemical methods in solution and biomedical applications. *Central European Journal of Chemistry* 2010;9(1):7–19.

[33] Hamidi M, Azadi A, Rafiei P. Hydrogel nanoparticles in drug delivery. *Advanced Drug Delivery Reviews* 2008;60(15):1638–1649.

[34] Zhang S, Ermann J, Succi MD, et al. An inflammation-targeting hydrogel for local drug delivery in inflammatory bowel disease. *Science Translational Medicine* 2015;7(300):300ra128.

[35] Hu R, Li G, Jiang Y, et al. Silver—zwitterion organic—inorganic nanocomposite with antimicrobial and antiadhesive capabilities. *Langmuir.* 2013;29(11):3773–3779.

[36] Lara HH, Ayala-Núñez NV, Padilla CR. Bactericidal effect of silver nanoparticles against multidrug-resistant bacteria. *World Journal of Microbiology and Biotechnology* 2010;26(4):615–621.

[37] Dallas P, Sharma VK, Zboril R. Silver polymeric nanocomposites as advanced antimicrobial agents: classification, synthetic paths, applications, and perspectives. Advances in Colloid and Interface Science 2011;166(1–2):119–135.

[38] Faoucher E, Nativo P, Black K, et al. In situ preparation of network forming gold nanoparticles in agarose hydrogels. *Chemical Communications* 2009;43:6661.

[39] Gong JP, Katsuyama Y, Kurokawa T, Osada Y. Double-network hydrogels with extremely high mechanical strength. *Advanced Materials* 2003;15:1155–1158.

[40] Peppas NA, Hilt JZ, Khademhosseini A, Langer R. Hydrogels in biology and medicine: from molecular principles to bionanotechnology. *Advanced Materials.* 2006;18:1345–1360.

[41] Hoffman AS. Hydrogels for biomedical applications. *Advanced Drug Delivery Reviews* 2002;54:3–12.

[42] Check E. Scientists rethink approach to HIV gels. *Nature.* 2007;446:12.

[43] Cheng SY, Heilman S, Wasserman M, Archer S, Shuler ML, Wu M. A hydrogel-based microfluidic device for the studies of directed cell migration. *Lab on a Chip.* 2007 **7**, 763–769.

[44] Nayak S, Lyon LA. Soft nanotechnology with soft nanoparticles. *Angewandte Chemie International Edition* 2005;44:7686–7708.

[45] Huh AJ, Kwon YJ. "Nanoantibiotics": a new paradigm for treating infectious diseases using nanomaterials in the antibiotics resistant era. *Journal of Controlled Release* 2011;156(2):128–145.

[46] Varghese S, Elisseeff JH. Hydrogels for musculoskeletal engineering. *Advances in Polymer Science* 2006;203:95–144.

[47] Drury JL, Mooney DJ. Hydrogels for tissue engineering: scaffold design variables and applications. *Biomaterials.* 2003;24:4337–4351.

[48] Dong L, Agarwal AK, Beebe DJ, Jiang H. Adaptive liquid microlenses activated by stimuli-responsive hydrogels. *Nature.* 2006;442:551–553.

[49] Hu R, Li G, Jiang Y, et al. Silver—zwitterion organic—inorganic nanocomposite with antimicrobial and antiadhesive capabilities. *Langmuir.* 2013;29(11):3773–3779.

[50] Ghobril C, Grinstaff MW. The chemistry and engineering of polymeric hydrogel adhesives for wound closure: a tutorial. *Chemical Society Reviews.* 2015;44(7): 1820–1835.

[51] Kozlovskaya V, Kharlampieva E, Chang S, Muhlbauer R, Tsukruk VV. pH-responsive layered hydrogel microcapsules as gold nanoreactors. *Chemistry of Materials* 2009;21(10):2158–2167.

[52] Guiney LM, Agnello AD, Thomas JC, Takatori K, Flynn NT. Thermoresponsive behavior of charged N-isopropylacrylamide-based hydrogels containing gold nanostructures. *Colloid and Polymer Science* 2009;287(5):601–608.

[53] Yalcinkaya F, Komarek M. Polyvinyl butyral (PVB) nanofiber/nanoparticle-covered yarns for antibacterial textile surfaces. *International Journal of Molecular Sciences.* 2019 Sep 3;20(17).

[54] Huang WS, Chu IM. Injectable polypeptide hydrogel/inorganic nanoparticle composites for bone tissue engineering. *PLoS One.* 2019;14(1):e0210285.

[55] Pasqui D, Atrei A, Giani G, De Cagna M, Barbucci R. Metal oxide nanoparticles as cross-linkers in polymeric hybrid hydrogels. *Materials Letters* 2011;65:392–395.

[56] Ahmed E.M. Hydrogel: preparation, characterization, and applications: a review. *Journal of Advanced Research* 2015;6:105–121.

[57] Neibert K, Gopishetty V, Grigoryev A, et al. Wound-healing with mechanically robust and biodegradable hydrogel fibers loaded with silver nanoparticles. *Advanced Healthcare Materials* 2012;1(5):621–630.

[58] Casero C, Machin F, Mendez-Alvarez S, et al. Structure and antimicrobial activity of phloroglucinol derivatives from *Achyrocline satureioides*. *Journal of Natural Products* 2015;78(1):93–102.

[59] Hosny KM. Ciprofloxacin as ocular liposomal hydrogel. *AAPS PharmSciTech.* 2010;11(1):241–246.

[60] Manju S, Antony M, Sreenivasan K. Synthesis and evaluation of a hydrogel that binds glucose and releases ciprofloxacin. *Journal of Materials Science* 2010;45(15):4006–4012.

[61] Shukla S and Shukla A. Tunable antibiotic delivery from gellanhydrogels. *Journal of Materials Chemistry B* 2018;6:6444–6458.

[62] Lakes AL, Peyyala R, Ebersole JL, Puleo DA, Hilt JZ, Dziubla TD. Synthesis and characterization of an antibacterial hydrogel containing covalently bound vancomycin. *Biomacromolecules.* 2014;15(8):3009–3018.

[63] Gustafson CT, Boakye-Agyeman F, Brinkman CL, et al. Controlled delivery of vancomycin via charged hydrogels. *PLoS One.* 2016;11(1):e0146401.

[64] Grohs P, Podglajen I, Guerot E, et al. Assessment of five screening strategies for optimal detection of carriers of third-generation cephalosporin-resistant Enterobacteriaceae in intensive care units using daily sampling. *Clinical Microbiology and Infection.* 2014;20(11):O879–O886.

[65] Lv ZF, Wang FC, Zheng HL, et al. Meta-analysis: is combination of tetracycline and amoxicillin suitable for *Helicobacter pylori* infection? *World Journal of Gastroenterology* 2015;21(8):2522–2533.

[66] Chang CH, Lin YH, Yeh CL, et al. Nanoparticles incorporated in pH-sensitive hydrogels as amoxicillin delivery for eradication of *Helicobacter pylori*. *Biomacromolecules.* 2010;11(1):133–142.

[67] Tormos CJ, Abraham C, Madihally SV. Improving the stability of chitosan-gelatin-based hydrogels for cell delivery using transglutaminase and controlled release of doxycycline. *Drug Delivery and Translational Research* 2015;5(6):575–584.

[68] Vergis J, Gokulakrishnan P, Agarwal RK, Kumar A. Essential oils as natural food antimicrobial agents: a review. *Critical Reviews in Food Science and Nutrition* 2015;55(10):1320–1323.

[69] Fan L, Yang J, Wu H, et al. Preparation and characterization of quaternary ammonium chitosan hydrogel with significant antibacterial activity. *International Journal of Biological Macromolecules* 2015;79:830–836.

[70] Brown AN, Smith K, Samuels TA, Lu J, Obare SO, Scott ME. Nanoparticles functionalized with ampicillin destroy multiple-antibiotic-resistant isolates of *Pseudomonas aeruginosa* and *Enterobacter aerogenes* and methicillin-resistant *Staphylococcus aureus*. *Applied and Environmental Microbiology* 2012;78(8):2768.

[71] Brogden KA. Antimicrobial peptides: pore formers or metabolic inhibitors in bacteria? *Nature Reviews Microbiology* 2005;3(3):238–250.

[72] Lakshmaiah Narayana J, Chen JY. Antimicrobial peptides: possible anti-infective agents. *Peptides.* 2015;72:88–94.

[73] Liu Y, Yang Y, Wang C, Zhao X. Stimuli-responsive self-assembling peptides made from antibacterial peptides. *Nanoscale.* 2013;5(14):6413–6421.

[74] Cleophas RT, Sjollema J, Busscher HJ, Kruijtzer JA, Liskamp RM. Characterization and activity of an immobilized antimicrobial peptide containing bactericidal PEG-hydrogel. *Biomacromolecules.* 2014;15(9):3390–3395.

[75] Pletzer D, Hancock RE. Antibiofilm peptides: potential as broad- spectrum agents. *Journal of Bacteriology* 2016;198(19):2572–2578.

[76] Nguyen, Tan Dat, et al. "In vivo study of the antibacterial chitosan/polyvinyl alcohol loaded with silver nanoparticle hydrogel for wound healing applications." *International Journal of Polymer Science*, (2019), 7382717 1-10.

[77] Abraham A, Soloman P, Rejini V. Preparation of chitosan-polyvinyl alcohol blends and studies on thermal and mechanical properties. *Procedia Technology* 2016;24:741–748.

[78] Zafar M, Shah T, Rawal A, Siores E. Preparation and characterisation of thermoresponsive nanogels for smart antibacterial fabrics. *Materials Science and Engineering C* 2014;40:135–141.

[79] Boonkaew B, Kempf M, Kimble R, Supaphol P, Cuttle L. Antimicrobial efficacy of a novel silver hydrogel dressing compared to two common silver burn wound dressings: acticoat and PolyMem Silver((R)). *Burns*. 2014;40(1):89–96.

[80] Simoes SM, Veiga F, Torres-Labandeira JJ, et al. Syringeable pluronicalpha-cyclodextrin supramolecular gels for sustained delivery of vancomycin. *European Journal of Pharmaceutics and Biopharmaceutics*, 2012;80(1):103–112.

[81] Pakzad Y, Ganji F. Thermosensitive hydrogel for periodontal application: in vitro drug release, antibacterial activity and toxicity evaluation. *Journal of Biomaterials Applications* 2016;30(7):919–929.

[82] Kong M, Chen XG, Xing K, Park HJ. Antimicrobial properties of chitosan and mode of action: a state of the art review. *International Journal of Food Microbiology* 2010;144(1):51–63.

[83] Mohamed RR, Seoudi RS, Sabaa MW. Synthesis and characterization of antibacterial semi-interpenetrating carboxymethyl chitosan/poly (acrylonitrile) hydrogels. *Cellulose*. 2012;19(3):947–958.

[84] Tsao CT, Chang CH, Lin YY, et al. Antibacterial activity and biocompatibility of a chitosan-gamma-poly(glutamic acid) polyelectrolyte complex hydrogel. *Carbohydrate Research* 2010;345(12):1774–1780.

[85] Chang HW, Lin YS, Tsai YD, Tsai ML. Effects of chitosan characteristics on the physicochemical properties, antibacterial activity, and cytotoxicity of chitosan/2-glycerophosphate/nanosilver hydrogels. *Journal of Applied Polymer Science* 2013;127(1):169–176.

[86] Guzman-Trampe S, Ceapa CD, Manzo-Ruiz M, Sanchez S. Synthetic biology era: improving antibiotic's world. *Biochemical Pharmacology* 2017;134:99–113.

[87] 166. Zhang J-Z, Xiao C-S, Wang J-C, Zhuang X-L, Chen X-S. Photo cross-linked biodegradable hydrogels for enhanced vancomycin loading and sustained release. *Chinese Journal of Polymer Science* 2013;31(12):1697–1705.

[88] Vaghani SS, Patel MM, Satish CS. Synthesis and characterization of pH-sensitive hydrogel composed of carboxymethyl chitosan for colon targeted delivery of ornidazole. *Carbohydrate Research* 2012;347(1):76–82.

[89] Das D, Ghosh P, Ghosh A, et al. Stimulus-responsive, biodegradable, biocompatible, covalently cross-linked hydrogel based on dextrin and Poly(N-isopropylacrylamide) for in vitro/in vivo controlled drug release. *ACS Applied Materials & Interfaces* 2015;7(26):14338–14351.

[90] Lboutounne H, Chaulet J-F, Ploton C, Falson F, Pirot F. Sustained ex vivo skin antiseptic activity of chlorhexidine in poly (ε-caprolactone) nanocapsule encapsulated form and as a digluconate. *Journal of Controlled Release* 2002;82(2):319–334.

10 Challenges and Future Prospects Associated with Smart Hydrogels for Drug Delivery and Imaging

Arti Vashist, Rameen Walters, and Madhavan Nair

CONTENTS

10.1 INTRODUCTION

In the past few decades, research on hydrogel technology has rapidly expanded due to its highly versatile and tunable characteristics [1–3]. Their hydrophilic nature allows them to absorb large amounts of water, swelling without compromising their structures and the tunable characteristic features. The smart hydrogels include the hydrogel system, which is developed in various forms such as nanogels [4, 5], hydrogel thin films, injectable gels, and nanocomposite hydrogels [6], and purposely introduced the smart properties such as they are made stimuli responsive [7]. Stimuli-responsive hydrogels are known to act smart depending on their properties [8]. Examples are pH-responsive hydrogels [9], magnetic hydrogels,

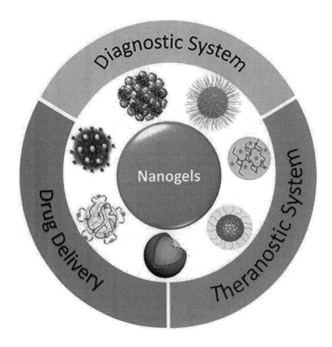

FIGURE 10.1   Hydrogels and nanogels for therapeutics and diagnostics.

Source: Reprinted with copyright permission (2016) from American Chemical Society [10].

pressure-responsive hydrogels, temperature-responsive hydrogels, etc. The various properties including physical, chemical, and mechanical features can be modulated depending on the diverse applications. Smart or stimuli-responsive hydrogels bear an additional property in their ability to alter their structure and function in response to a specific environmental trigger. The variety of smart hydrogels utilize temperature, pH, electric or magnetic fields, light, and biomolecular or chemical triggers [1, 2]. While the variety of smart hydrogel formulations that have been developed are vast and continually growing, they are not without their challenges and limitations. Several general factors are important when considering the development of hydrogels or nanogels for diagnostic or therapeutic (Figure 10.1) use including biocompatibility, mechanical strength, size, and shape, among other factors. In this chapter, the challenges and limitations of smart hydrogel technologies will be discussed along with its future prospects.

10.2   CHALLENGES AND LIMITATIONS OF SMART HYDROGELS

The present section will discuss in detail the limitations and challenges imposed by smart hydrogel systems with respect to the biocompatibility, mechanical strength, size, methods of drying, route of administrations, and responsive features of the hydrogels.

10.2.1 BIOCOMPATIBILITY AND MECHANICAL STRENGTH

Hydrogel composition is greatly varied, which is warranted by the broad selection of polymers to choose from. As a whole, hydrogel polymers can be classified into two categories: natural and synthetic. Natural polymers, such as chitosan [3], hyaluronan [4], collagen [4], alginates [11], and fibrin [12], are often considered the most viable options for diagnostic and therapeutic uses. This viability is attributed to the non-toxic, biodegradable nature of these polymers; however, they do come with some inherent limitations. Sterility and reproducibility are a concern when using these hydrogels since they come from natural sources. This may be attributed to the inability to control the composition of different batches of a natural product. The more profound limitation of natural hydrogels is their lack of mechanical strength and stability. To supplement this limitation, other polymers and crosslinking agents may be added to the formulation of the hydrogel to try to strengthen the gels, with synthetic additives potentially being considered for this purpose. Synthetic hydrogels are made up of materials such as polyethylene glycol diacrylate, polyacrylamide, and polyvinyl alcohol [13]. These synthetic polymers will add the necessary strength to a natural hydrogel to stabilize it; however, while synthetic polymer composition and stability are easier to control and reproduce, they will often increase the toxicity of the gel. Developing a suitable hydrogel for therapeutic or diagnostic purposes involves balancing the use of natural and synthetic polymers and finding the optimal level of stability and biocompatibility. The ultimate goal is to develop a hydrogel system that is stable enough to complete the task it is designed to perform while also capable of being degraded and removed from the body safely. For example, a recent interesting study by Chen et al. [14] showed the development of thermosensitive hydrogels used for local drug delivery which could reduce systemic toxicity and degrade in a three-week time period. Figure 10.2 shows that the hydrogels, when incubated with enzyme, showed higher weight loss. In the presence of Proteinase K, the gel disappeared, and in the presence of elastase, 85% of mass loss was observed.

10.2.2 SIZE

Particle size is an important factor in hydrogel development, particularly with micro/nanogel drug delivery systems, but it can be a challenge to control. In confluence with the previously discussed components of the hydrogel, size tends to play a role in the biocompatibility/biodegradability of a hydrogel. Size must be considered when designing a system that will travel through the human body. Studies have shown that hydrogels <200 nm in diameter can go through the spleen and those that are <20 nm can be excreted through the kidneys [7]. Size must be considered when designing a delivery system to areas of the body that are difficult to access such as the brain. The challenge of producing hydrogels of a particular size may be overcome using a variety of methods [15]. Several techniques can be utilized to generate hydrogel particles, each with its size variations. The use of the emulsion technique tends to produce polydisperse micro- and nano-sized particles whereas ionic gelation generates homogeneous suspended nano-sized particles [16]. Depending on the method of gel formulation, increases in stirring speed and time of the suspended forming particles will lead to a

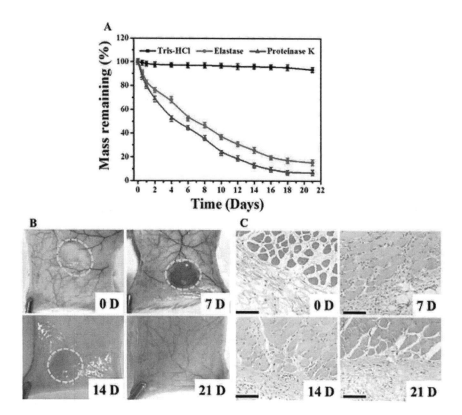

FIGURE 10.2 (A) In vitro mass loss profiles for the in situ formed mPEG45-PELG12 (6 wt%) hydrogels incubated in Tris-HCl buffer (0.05 M, pH 7.4) containing 5 U/ml−1 proteinase K or elastase and Tris-HCl buffer without enzyme as control. (B) In situ gel formation and in vivo gel maintenance. mPEG45-PELG12 solutions (0.5 ml, 8 wt%) were subcutaneously injected in the back of rats. Photos around the implants (marked as yellow-dotted curves) were taken 30 min (0 day), 7, 14, and 21 days after the injection. (C) Histological images of the subcutaneous tissues surrounding the hydrogels (H & E staining). Scale bar = 100 μm. (For interpretation of the references to color in this figure caption, the reader is referred to the web version of this chapter.)

Source: Reprinted with copyright permission (2016) from American Chemical Society [14].

smaller particle likely caused by the shearing forces of said stirring [17]. Dried particles can be crushed and subsequently sorted using sets of fine meshes or filters with decreasingly small pores. This technique will reduce the size of the final product but will result in a decreased yield and a variable polydispersity index (PDI) [18]. Recently, high-frequency sonication, such as probe sonication, has been utilized for particle shrinkage. Sonication will break apart the gel into smaller particles; however, this can come with some caveats. The heat generated by the sonication may be detrimental to the structure and characteristics of the hydrogel if left unchecked. In order to mitigate the problems caused by excess heat, the hydrogel solution can be placed in cold water or ice bath during sonication [19]. Given the hydrophilic nature of hydrogels, they also tend to swell within an aqueous medium. Modulation of swelling can be done by adding hydrophobic moieties, such as linseed oil–derived polyol, to the particle solution during its formation.

10.2.3 DRYING

Stable hydrogels are capable of preserving their structure and functionality for very long periods, which provides hydrogel products a lengthy shelf life. This is one of the lures of using hydrogels; however, obtaining a dried product from hydrogels suspended in a solution can pose a challenge.

10.2.4 ROUTE OF ADMINISTRATION

In the clinical setting, the diagnostic or therapeutic application of smart hydrogels can take many forms: micro/nanoparticles, coatings, films, and slabs. This is the matchless property of these soft materials that they can be formed in various shapes. These unparalleled characteristics keep them apart from all existing drug delivery systems. These gels have been utilized in developing everything from contacts to diapers. Smart hydrogels, in their various forms, may take advantage of various routes of administration, each with its own set of challenges. Hydrogels are often given through oral means due to their easy access and the protection of the gel's contents against liver enzymes [20]. However, oral routes of administration have the innate challenge of overcoming the pH variability within the digestive system, particularly the acidic environment of the stomach. The potential instability of a gel within acidic environments must be overcome to establish a viable oral route of distribution. For example, the premature release of a drug and degradation of the hydrogel may be a challenge in a pH-sensitive delivery system that could perhaps take advantage of the low pH tumor environment [1]. Intranasal administration of hydrogels may be used to take advantage of the quick access to the brain through the olfactory cranial nerves. The challenge in using this route is that it is size dependent, with smaller particles being the most effective.

10.2.5 STIMULI SENSITIVITY

The external factors largely influence the characteristic properties of hydrogels. These external factors are the key to the unique specificity achieved using hydrogel for therapeutics and diagnostics. Table 10.1 represents some of the common challenges associated with the various stimuli-responsive hydrogels used for various biomedical applications.

It is very imperative to recognize the functional behavior of hydrogels, and thus we can utilize the stimuli-responsive nature for on-demand drug delivery or active targeting of the drugs.

TABLE 10.1

Challenges of Producing a Smart Hydrogel That Has Optimal Sensitivity

Temperature-sensitive hydrogels	• The critical point, or the temperature at which gelation occurs, decreases as polymer size increases [2].
	• Synthetic polymers have fast responses whereas natural polymers, which are preferred for biocompatibility, have limited response at physiological temperatures [2].
Photosensitive hydrogels (UV)	• Ultraviolet light does not penetrate deep into the body, which limits the capabilities of these hydrogels.

10.3 FUTURE PROSPECTS

The future of smart hydrogels is one of great promise. The applications of hydrogels are already greatly varied, from drug delivery to biosensing to wound healing. Overcoming the challenges posed by different kinds of hydrogels will, of course, be a large part of future research. Further optimization and specialization of the different aspects of hydrogel applications will be a major part of this research. Hydrogel delivery systems are still in the fairly early stages of development and are venturing into new territory, including drug delivery to the central nervous system, gene delivery, and tissue engineering.

10.3.1 THE BLOOD-BRAIN BARRIER

As the mean age of the population continues to rise, occurrences of various neurodegenerative disorders rise with it. This increase in neurologic disease rates, concurrently with the recent heightened interest in mental health, has led to a push for more research on the brain and how it can be influenced. One major challenge in this field has been the restriction of using therapies that are unable to bypass the blood-brain barrier (BBB). Future smart hydrogels [21] will likely be able to navigate, guided by chemical or magnetic signals, and perform delivery or healing functions in the brain (Figure 10.3).

10.3.2 GENE DELIVERY

With the recent advent of the CRISPR/Cas9 genomic editing system, a variety of delivery systems have been explored, with hydrogels providing an excellent option for a myriad of reasons. Hydrogels, due to their structure, are capable of improving the stability of incorporated macromolecules such as the Cas9 protein. This way it maintains the editing efficiency of Cas9 while providing a method of maximizing the specificity of its targeting, which minimizes the undesired effects of constitutively active Cas9.

There are other gene delivery methods, generally used in cancer therapy, that involve the use of hydrogels. Smart hydrogels can be used to encapsulate siRNAs or lethal DNA genes and sent them to a target cell to promote apoptosis [20].

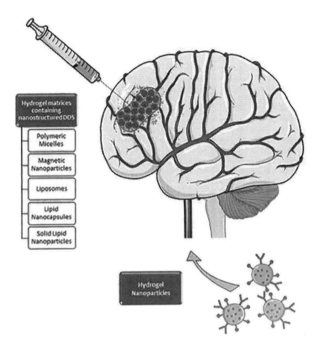

FIGURE 10.3   Hydrogel nanoparticle potential candidate for the treatment of brain tumors.

Source: Reprinted with copyright permission (2018) from Molecular Diversity Preservation International and Multidisciplinary Digital Publishing Institute (MDPI Pulishers) [22].

10.3.3   Tissue Engineering and Bioprinting

The use of hydrogels for wound healing and tissue regeneration has been well docu-mented, and the natural progression of such technologies would involve tissue engi-neering and bioprinting. In wound healing, hydrogels behave a scaffolds for cells to grow along. The hydrogels contain nutrients and growth factors to maintain cell proliferation. In tissue engineering, smart hydrogels may hold various tools to spe-cialize and grow tissues or even organs. There have been recent studies looking at the use of hydrogels to develop tissue that could be used to repair damaged cardiac tissue. In these studies, electrically conductive hydrogels were used as scaffolds to grow cardiac cells [23].

10.3.4   Cancer Immunotherapy

One of the primary issues that has captured the minds of the scientific community has been the delivery of therapeutic agents to specific cancerous tissues. The limita-tions related to many of the current therapeutic options relate to toxicity, prolonged drug activity, and specificity. The most tedious aspects to be addressed are the com-plexities and instabilities of present drug delivery technology associated with a lack of specificity, meaning the therapies attack "off-targets," such as normal tissues. In recent years, cancer immunotherapy has received a considerable amount of attention due to its unique ability to boost the immune system to target and destroy cancer cells and prevent recurrence in the long term. This contrasts starkly with many chemotherapies that function by targeting rapidly dividing cells, which, in turn, compromises the bone marrow and thus the immune system. These new immunotherapies include immune checkpoint inhibitors, cancer vaccines, other macromolecular drugs (such as cytokines and antibodies), and the chimeric antigen receptor T (CAR-T) cells [24]. Many of these incredible new therapies do have limitations, such as rapid elimination by reticuloendothelial systems and high interstitial fluid pressures within tumors. They also have drawbacks due to their systemic administration such as the requirement of high doses, numerous injections, and the development of severe side effects like autoimmune disease. While immunotherapy is generally more specific than many of the other therapeutic options, systemic administration can be harmful. The utilization of smart hydrogels can address these obstacles. The use of pH- and ROS (reactive oxygen species)- responsive hydrogels could take advantage of tumor microenvironments and administer therapies locally by providing a specifically targeted method of delivery.

10.4   CONCLUSIONS

The diverse applications of hydrogel technology and the ease of development of these smart materials make them a potential candidate to explore further for future development. Their resemblance to the extracellular matrix makes them highly compatible with the human system. The major focus of emerging research is to combat present limitations and challenges associated with existing hydrogel systems. Still, we have to overcome the toxicity accompanying these smart materials. There is an immense need to explore hydrogels at nanoscale, which can improve the limitations of existing nanodelivery vehicles and address the existing challenges.

10.5   CONFLICT OF INTEREST

The authors declare no conflict of interest.

10.6   ACKNOWLEDGMENTS

The authors acknowledge the financial support from the National Institute of Health (NIH) grants 1R01DA037838–01, 1R01DA040537–01, and R01DA034547.

REFERENCES

[1] A. Vashist, A. Kaushik, A. Vashist, J. Bala, R. Nikkhah-Moshaie, V. Sagar, M. Nair, Nanogels as potential drug nanocarriers for CNS drug delivery, *Drug Discovery Today*, 23 (2018) 1436–1443.

[2] O. Erol, A. Pantula, W. Liu, D.H. Gracias, Transformer hydrogels: A review, *Advanced Materials Technologies*, 4 (2019) 1900043.

[3] A. Vashist, A. Vashist, Y. Gupta, S. Ahmad, Recent advances in hydrogel based drug delivery systems for the human body, *Journal of Materials Chemistry B*, 2 (2014) 147–166.

[4]   A. Vashist, A. Kaushik, A. Ghosal, R. Nikkhah-Moshaie, A. Vashist, R. Dev Jayant, M. Nair, Chapter 1 journey of hydrogels to nanogels: A decade after, in: *Nanogels for Biomedical Applications*, The Royal Society of Chemistry, 2018, pp. 1–8.

[5]   A. Ghosal, S. Tiwari, A. Mishra, A. Vashist, N.K. Rawat, S. Ahmad, J. Bhattacharya, Design and engineering of nanogels, in: *Nanogels for Biomedical Applications*, RSC publishers 2017, pp. 9–28.

[6]   A. Vashist, A. Kaushik, A. Ghosal, J. Bala, R. Nikkhah-Moshaie, W.A. Wani, P. Manickam, M. Nair, Nanocomposite hydrogels: Advances in nanofillers used for nano-medicine, *Gels*, 4 (2018) 75.

[7]   A. Vashist, A. Kaushik, K. Alexis, J.R. Dev, V. Sagar, A. Vashist, M. Nair, Bioresponsive injectable hydrogels for on-demand drug release and tissue engineering, *Current Pharmaceutical Design*, 23 (2017) 3595.

[8]   A. Ghosal, A. Vashist, S. Tiwari, A. Kaushik, R.D. Jayant, M. Nair, J. Bhattacharya, Hydrogels: Smart nanomaterials for biomedical applications, in: *Synthesis of Inorganic Nanomaterials*, Elsevier, 2018, pp. 283–292.

[9]   R. Kouser, A. Vashist, M. Zafaryab, M.A. Rizvi, S. Ahmad, pH-Responsive bio-compatible nanocomposite hydrogels for therapeutic drug delivery, *ACS Applied Bio Materials*, 1 (2018) 1810–1822.

[10] H-Q. Wu, C-C. Wang, Biodegradable smart nanogels: A new platform for targeting drug delivery and biomedical diagnostics, *Langmuir*, 32 (2016) 6211–6225.

[11] Y. Zhang, X. Li, N. Zhong, Y. Huang, K. He, X. Ye, Injectable in situ dual-crosslink-ing hyaluronic acid and sodium alginate based hydrogels for drug release, *Journal of Biomaterials Science, Polymer Edition* (2019) 1–10.

[12] J.P. Garcia, J. Stein, Y. Cai, F. Riemers, E. Wexselblatt, J. Wengel, M. Tryfonidou, A. Yayon, K.A. Howard, L.B. Creemers, Fibrin-hyaluronic acid hydrogel-based delivery of antisense oligonucleotides for ADAMTS5 inhibition in co-delivered and resident joint cells in osteoarthritis, *Journal of Controlled Release*, 294 (2019) 247–258.

[13] F.M. Croisfelt, L.L. Tundisi, J.A. Ataide, E. Silveira, E.B. Tambourgi, A.F. Jozala, E.M.B. Souto, P.G. Mazzola, Modified-release topical hydrogels: A ten-year review, *Journal of Materials Science* (2019) 1–21.

[14] X. Wu, Y. Wu, H. Ye, S. Yu, C. He, X. Chen, Interleukin-15 and cisplatin co-encap-sulated thermosensitive polypeptide hydrogels for combined immuno-chemotherapy, *Journal of Controlled Release*, 255 (2017) 81–93.

[15] H.L. Lim, Y. Hwang, M. Kar, S. Varghese, Smart hydrogels as functional biomimetic systems, *Biomaterials Science*, 2 (2014) 603–618.

[16] N. Ferreira, L. Ferreira, V. Cardoso, F. Boni, A. Souza, M. Gremião, Recent advances in smart hydrogels for biomedical applications: From self-assembly to functional approaches, *European Polymer Journal*, 99 (2018) 117–133.

[17] A. Vashist, A. Kaushik, M. Nair, Micro/nano magnetic hydrogels with autofluores-cence for therapeutic and diagnostic applications, in, US Patent App. 15/907,703, 2019.

[18] S. Rother, V. Krönert, N. Hauck, A. Berg, S. Moeller, M. Schnabelrauch, J. Thiele, D. Scharnweber, V. Hintze, Hyaluronan/collagen hydrogel matrices containing high-sulfated hyaluronan microgels for regulating transforming growth factor-β1, *Journal of Materials Science: Materials in Medicine*, 30 (2019) 65.

[19] N. Chirani, L. Gritsch, F.L. Motta, S. Fare, History and applications of hydrogels, *Journal of Biomedical Sciences*, 4 (2015).

[20] P. Ghasemiyeh, S. Mohammadi-Samani, Hydrogels as drug delivery systems: Pros and Cons, *Trends in Pharmaceutical Sciences*, 5 (2019) 7–24.

[21] A. Vashist, A. Kaushik, J. Bala, H. Unwalla, V. Bhardwaj, V. Sagar, M. Nair, Nanogels for brain drug delivery, in: *Nanogels for Biomedical Applications*, RSC 2017, pp. 94–108.

[22] J. Basso, A. Miranda, S. Nunes, T. Cova, J. Sousa, C. Vitorino, A. Pais, Hydrogel-based drug delivery nanosystems for the treatment of brain tumors, *Gels*, 4 (2018) 62.

Index

Note: Page numbers in *italic* indicate a figure and page numbers in **bold** indicate a table on the corresponding page.

Printed and bound by CPI Group (UK) Ltd, Croydon, CR0 4YY

17/10/2024

01775681-0018